I0420982

CONGRATULATIONS

BACK TO

GOOD HEALTH

& Long Life

Amazon Press
2015

I write a column every week for a local newspaper

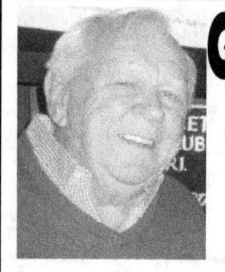

GETTING OLD-ER

You don't stop laughing because you grow old
You grow old because you stop laughing

by Jack Daly

STAY HEALTHY AND ENJOY LIFE

I'm kinda confirmed with "getting older" because it't better than the other option, which is dead!! So I'll take getting older.
Age-liars and birthday-deniers... you'd best learn a thing or two from me who is young at heart. I feel much younger than my actual chronological age.

Perceived age might play a role in more than just how you feel. I suggest it could be that those who feel "young at heart" have healthier behaviors and more resilience, giving them a stronger will to live. The good news is, you can change your perception of how young you are by keeping yourself in good shape by exercising every day.

When I got sick, I was told that I had to exercise to get better. That suggestion came from a good friend who explained that working out every day to get my body in good shape would be what I needed.

column not continued

TABLE OF CONTENTS

Introduction   page 1
Chapter 1
Getting Older Club   page 7
Chapter 2
Good Nutrition   page 11
Chapter 3
Living a Dream   page 15
Chapter 4
Aging Gracefully   page 23
Chapter 5
Enjoy a gift of a new day   page 29
Chapter 6
Working out   page 33
Chapter 7
All those aches and pains   page 41
Chapter 8
Sex, Intimacy and Companionship   page 47
Chapter 9
The No Strees Life   page 53
Chapter 10
The Joy of Volunteering ....   .page 57
Chapter 11
Nothing To Do & No Place To Go   page 59
Chapter 12
Age Liars and Birthday Deniers   page 69
Chapter 13
Healthy Aging   page 77

HOW DARE I WRITE THIS BOOK

It's true, I don't possess a Ph.D. So what gives me the authority to write this book? I am not a doctor, nutritionist, therapist or any sort of medical professional, but I felt compelled to write about my journey back to good health. I spent endless hours speaking with professionals, scouring my local library and researching various topics for this book on the Internet. I now know more about what happened to my body, and what makes a body tick, than I probably ever wanted to know. I've taken what I have learned and made it easily understandable to my readers. No big words, no fancy medical terms...just plain language.

ACKNOWLEDGMENTS

I thank the many and varied sources available in the public domain on the Internet. The availability of this technical research information was exactly what I needed to allow my readers to grasp the seriousness of maintaining good health.

I thank friends and, again, the Internet for the many great jokes liberally sprinkled throughout this work. My feeling is they added levity to an otherwise (could be) dull and complicated work.

I sincerely and passionately thank my dear, dear Annette for tireless support and countless hours of meticulous editing. She may never admit to being the power behind the throne, but she is!

Lastly, I thank Mike Bisceglia for making my words and thoughts much more interesting than I could ever have expressed.

.

Book Cover designed by DALY PHOTO
Hampton NH 03842
603-601-2733

WARNING
LAUGH YOUR WAY
BACK TO
GOOD HEALTH
Scattered throughout
this book are some
of the funniest jokes,
stories, antedotes, etc.
deliberately placed
between chapters
for the reader to
enjoy a little humor
amid the seriousness
of understanding
more about sickness
and good health.

INTRODUCTION

How my near-death experience brought about the birth of this book.

I had not been paying attention to my health; it was as simple as that. In recent years, I had been doing all of the wrong things and had been expecting my body to perform at maximum efficiency. It only goes to prove that age and wisdom do not necessarily go hand in hand.

My COPD flare-ups had been happening with more and more frequency. I was feeling completely rundown and disinterested in life. Frankly, I thought it was checkout time and I was about to turn in my key.

About lunch time one day, I had the good sense to call my close friend, Mike, to take me to the emergency room at a local hospital. He was at my home in seconds, and the look on his face indicated to me that this drive just might be my last. I was gasping for breath. I was soaked in sweat. I ached everywhere, and my heart was racing. I was a mess.

Amazingly, the folks at the check-in desk took one look at me and had me whisked into an examination room. My guess is that within two minutes someone must have shot out to tell Mike that I was to be admitted.

I had become the less-than-proud owner of a case of pneumonia. The prognosis was not enchanting due to the fact that the pneumonia had compromised my COPD. In a nutshell, my ability to breathe was nearly at an end. It was amazing how much I had taken the simple task of breathing for granted when I found I was not able to do it.

Even the simple act of walking across the room caused me unimaginable stress. A journey of a few feet simply wore me out. It was as though I had just raced a marathon at top speed.

They tried everything to control the pneumonia and to get me to breathe normally. After three weeks in the hospital, you can only imagine my feeling when I was informed that I would be needing a wheelchair and an oxygen tank as my constant companions. In addition, I had to make regular visits at a local rehab facility plus the intensive care I was to receive in my home from visiting nurses and therapists.

This routine went on for three months after the hospital discharge.. The visiting pulmonary therapist (PT) and the nurse managed to get me to walk an incredible 30 feet. . . . a personal best after two months of therapy. We celebrated! It was the best I could do before collapsing.

I was constantly monitoring myself with my oximeter to see if I was getting better. My oxygen reading was still at 84%, when it should have been reading 98%. I required the use of 100% oxygen for survival round the clock. All indications were that I was to be married to that cursed tank for the remainder of my life. In addition, my strength continued to deteriorate. It was the bottom of the ninth, and it certainly didn't look good for the home team.

Then, a remarkable thing happened just when I believed all hope was gone. A close friend came to visit with a message and a good idea. In short order, he presented every reason for me to begin an aggressive program of both vigorous exercise and quality nutrition. He said it would really get me out of the wheelchair and back to the land of the living. At first I cursed him because my body and mind never did like exercise, and I had never cared to pay any attention to nutrition, but in short order I began to make progress . . . real progress. In three months, after following his directions, I did more of the required exercises every day,

Soon after, I had no need for the oxygen tank and I was walking. My oxygen reading was normal and I could walk a mile on the beach with absolutely no discomfort thanks to Steve.

In the course of my campaign to become new and improved, I decided to write this book to make readers aware that they can live longer and happier lives...if they stay healthy.

The critical factor to begin this life-changing feat is sincerity and dedication to a good health goal and to start treating your body with some respect. You have to be sincere with yourself when you evaluate what you eat and how much you exercise. You have to honestly accept that once you choose to change your life that you make the commitment to stick to the program.

I grant you that facing the prospect of making changes to your current lifestyle may present a challenge, but you will see and feel the results very quickly depending how bad off you are.

I am not a doctor or any kind of a specialist on good health and nutrition. I am a prior newspaper editor/publisher telling a story of the amazing process of my survival while discovering the route back to good health. Good Nutrition, Aging Gracefully, All those Aches & Pains, Gift of a New Day, Sex, Intimacy & Companionship are just a few very interesting story lines in the book.

SICKNESS CHANGED MY LIFE.

I was so sick that the doctors and I were convinced I was going to die. I was hospitalized and given massive doses of God-knows-what' and I was preparing myself for the end,.I believed that I would not have long to wait.   Shortly, however, something amazing happened. With the love and care of some wonderful people I managed to live. Let there be no misunderstanding, when I was released from the hospital, I thought I was going home to die. I was being wheeled out of the hospital in a wheelchair equipped with an oxygen tank. I was wearing the mask and sucking in the breath of life. In my left arm an intravenous hook-up was providing me wit needed medication and sustenance.

In my right hand were the doctor's written orders. Essentially, he had spelled out that the lifestyle I was experiencing at that moment was exactly the lifestyle I would have for the rest of my abridged life span. There was no mention of any hope for recuperation. I was to drag that oxygen tank with me to the bathroom and back, and I could expect to be winded on both legs of the journey . . . a journey of no more than fifteen feet.

I mentioned "love and care by some wonderful people." Well, not all of it was of the kind and gentle variety. Some of my friends might have been better suited as Marine drill sergeants at Paris Island. They offered tough love and plenty of it. They told me that if I wanted to live . . . really, truly wanted to live, I was going to have to work, and I was going to have to stop being the pansy that led me to the condition I currently found myself in.

HEALING

My golfing buddy and best friend may actually have been an angel sent by God. He put his face directly in front of mine so I couldn't miss it, and he began to tell the affects that exercise and nutrition would have on my body. When he finished touting the praises of the stationary bike, he began to expound on the virtues of good eating habits. In guy terms, he essentially told me to get my ass off of that wheelchair and start a real, honest-to-god program of exercise and good eating habits. This program would include plenty of walking and a total daily beer intake of zero ounces of the amber-colored nectar of the gods. Oh, and one more little thing, this terrific package program was not a short term event. It was about to be my plan for the rest of my hoped-to-be very long life.

I laughed and asked him if he was kidding. He said that he was as serious as a heart attack. I stopped laughing and sighed. I had a very high mountain to climb, and I had only myself to blame.

I even joined a gym and actually go there religiously. I have cut down on my drinking (no mean fete for this Irishman). I walk. I meet people. And, more importantly, I think. I think of a future of feeling good. I think of what new and exciting adventures I can become involved in. I think of my next vacation. I think of the special times I could have with the ones I love. And, more importantly, I am now thinking of how to get better. It works!

I can't begin to thank all of the folks who pitched in when I was down for the count. They really rallied round me and lovingly kicked my ass. They truly didn't want me to check out . . . and, I do become choked up when I consider all that my merry band of friends did (and put up with) just to have this old coot stay alive and well. I'm not going to name names here, but suffice to say that all of you are in my heart . . . not necessarily in my will! . . . an email or two would pop up on my screen, and I would know that people still care. In reality, I'm sure I knew that I had caring people in my life. I guess my amazement is the depth of their concern. I would only hope that if the tables were reversed, could I match the concern they have shown for me. With God's grace, I would.

I SOLD MY BUSINESS

Because of my near death experience, there seemed no other way out. I made a decision that caused me no small degree of consternation. I sold my newspaper business. This reality, coupled with my failing health, plunged me into an abyss of depression. My newspaper had been my child. I had brought it into the world . . . and now it was gone. I felt like crying all of the time.   .

"My memory is gone, Mildred, so I changed my password to "Incorrect." That way when I log in with the wrong password, the computer will tell me... "Your password is incorrect."

"My doctor gave me six months to live. I couldn't pay the bill, so he gave me another six months.

That's for 40 years of lousy sex!'

An elderly couple was sitting quietly on the porch in their rocking chairs when the old man suddenly reached across and slapped his wife in the face. 'What was that for?' she demanded. 'That's for 40 years of lousy sex!'

She didn't say anything, but a few minutes later she slapped him back. 'What was that for?' he cried. 'That's for knowing the difference!'"

Late Night Lecture

An elderly man driving erratically was stopped by the police around 2 a.m. and was asked where he was going at that time of night.

The man replied, "I'm on my way to a lecture about alcohol abuse and the effects it has on the human body, as well as smoking and staying out late."

The officer then asked, "Really? Who's giving that lecture at this time of night?"

The man replied, "That would be my wife.

CHAPTER 1

GETTING OLDER CLUB

You must be physically able and willing to do things . . . walk, climb stairs, play sports, and have sex, etc.

A simple truth here . . . each of us is going to age. It is going to happen at lightning speed. You won't see it coming. You'll just be living your life the way you always have, thinking, I sure am young! There is little in life that I enjoy more than the simple knowledge of how completely not old I am. And then one day, out of the blue, you'll have a horrifying realization that people have stopped viewing you as an ultra cool, iconic masterpiece of sexuality ... now you're just another old guy.

I'm almost certain that my first tip-off came when a sales-clerk at a local grocery called me "sir." In a day or two, I spotted my first grey hair. That night, that hair extended an invitation to all of his friends. The next day, I had grey hair everywhere!

It is curious just how the definition of "old" varies according to the speaker. At 84, young people in their 20's see me as an old guy. If I were to talk to someone in his 70's, I would be considered young. I joke about being an old man, but Peter Pan and I have something in common . . . both of us refuse to grow up!

Remember, there are requirements to the "getting older club". You must be physically able and willing to do things . . . walk, climb stairs, play sports, and have sex, etc. To want to feel good about yourself is absolutely and completely up to you! Me? I get bored easily when I find nothing interesting to do. When that happens, I go to a health facility. I go at least once a day every day to work out for an hour or so. At 84, this old body hurts when I walk and exercise, but the idea that I'm off to the gym really does make me feel good. Later, after I've showered and tossed my sweaty gym clothes in my bag, I am delighted that I went. I feel exhilarated and ready for whatever the rest of the day has to offer. I might be hurting, but it usually is a good hurt.

Before you begin to believe that I'm some kind of geriatric superman, please allow me to be perfectly honest. When I began my exercise program, all those exercises and pedalling (but going nowhere) . . . I hated every *&^%$#@ moment. My legs killed me. I suffered with every step. All I wanted to do was to live it up and relax. I had to convince myself that what I was doing was good for me. I needed a new mind set.

Make no mistake about it, it was a tough time for this old man. I was stuck in the worst New Hampshire winter on record, and all I wanted to do was to sip umbrella drinks poolside in Florida. I didn't keep a log, (frankly, I thought I wouldn't be alive long enough to make that venture worthwhile) but that month was brutal. About the point I thought I would throw in the towel, some chemical in my body kicked in. I began to like the new routine. I got up to an hour of fast-pedalling and a mile on the treadmill. I had some upper body exercises and managed a short walk in the cold sun. Needless to say, I did more than survive; I thrived!

. I also like to play computer games on the Internet now that I'm retired from the newspaper biz. I'm glued to the computer screen for hours on end playing duplicate bridge. That keeps me happy for a very, very long time. My lady friend also plays her style of games on an adjoining computer and we both enjoying ourselves. We did at least an hour of exercise and/ or walking earlier in the day and now we feel comfortable just relaxing and doing what so ever we want.

"I'm not someone who thrives on a lot of unscripted time.

I like the feeling that there is still time for me to grow and time for a possible new business venture (adventure) and new things to do. Writing a column for my old paper the Seacoast Scene is one of them. I still have all of my mental faculties. My health is good and I still have the urgency to get things done. I feel vital, and that's all that matters.

All that I have described in this chapter and throughout this book works for me. My exercise regimen, my diet, and my social life work very well for me. Moreover, I want to be in good health to enjoy good food, my time at the gym and my friends and family. My health and wellbeing are mutually dependent upon one another. When I let my health slide, I was unwittingly lessening those items I really enjoy and shortening my time upon this earth. It is really a very simple equation when you stop to think about it.

Are you ready? Okay . . . STOP! Now, think about it (it, of course being a longer, healthier and happier life). Did you find yourself making a commitment to becoming a happier, healthier you? You should have. Here's a sad fact, gym enrolments rocket skyward every year just prior to New Year's Eve. Enrollment drops off dramatically by the end of January.

Okay, here comes the tough love. No one is going to take you by the hand to help you along through this journey of life. That's your job. No one is going to stick a star on your forehead or pat you on the back each time you do the right thing. Conversely, not many folks are going to be kind enough to let you know when you're not doing so well either. Consider this book to be your wake-up call.

Don't fall for the myth that growing older automatically means you're not going to feel good anymore.

It is true that aging involves physical changes, but it doesn't have to mean discomfort and disability. While not all illness or pain is avoidable, many of the physical challenges associated with aging can be overcome by eating right, exercising, and taking care of yourself.

One of the most important things you can do to stay healthy in your golden years is to **maintain your sense of purpose** by staying connected to people and things that matter to you. However, this isn't always easy—especially in a society that all-too-often views older people as a burden.

Quote from his chapter

"When I let my health slide, I was unwittingly lessening those itimes I really enjoyed and shortening my time upon this earth. It is really a very simple equation when you stop to think about it".

"Do you think I'll live to be 90?"

I recently picked a new primary care doctor. After two visits and exhaustive lab tests, he said I was doing "fairly well" for my age. A little concerned about that comment,I couldn't resist asking him, "Do you think I'll live to be 90?" He asked, "Do you smoke tobacco, or drink beer or wine?" "Oh no," I replied. "I'm not doing drugs, either. "Then he asked, "Do you eat rib-eye steaks and barbecued ribs?"I said, "No, my former doctor said that all red meat is very unhealthy!" "Do you spend a lot of time in the sun, like playing golf, sailing, hiking, or bicycling?""No I don't," I said He asked, "Do you gamble, drive fast cars, or have a lot of sex?" "No," I said. "I don't do any of those things. He looked at me and said, "Then, why do you care?"

Processed food is unhealthy. If it looks like it was made in a factory, don't eat it.

CHAPTER 2

GOOD NUTRITION
"YA GOTTA EAT RIGHT!!"

If you want to stay healthy, you better start eating right and stop eating foods that are going to hurt you

It is a fact. The food system has become more and more technologically perfect, but the general health of America's population has grossly deteriorated. Simply put, during food processing, many of the beneficial nutrients, which should be contained in the foods are either removed or have been greatly reduced and are replaced by any number of additives. Sadly, consumers purchase foods at the supermarket in the belief that they are doing right for their families and themselves. In reality, just the reverse may be true. Thus, eating to stay healthy in this day and age is a constant and arduous struggle.

Okay, back to basics. Good nutrition is essential to maintaining good health. The subject of nutrition is very complex . probably more so than need be. In this chapter, I will attempt to tackle only the main issues necessary to stay healthy. Let's dig in, shall we?

1.Let's get real. The most important thing you can do to ensure optimal health is to eat real food. Food supplements are not real foods. They are not able to replace the nutrients a body needs to function normally.

2. Processed foods are not necessarily unhealthy, but they may just be empty. The word, "processed" is perfectly stated. Processed foods are chemically or genetically produced in hot house gardens or factories. They are designed to be fast-growing, and, perhaps, smell and taste like their natural counterparts, but don't be fooled . . . they do bodies more harm than good. A simple rule of thumb here: If it looks like it was made in a factory, don't eat it.

Stress eating is not an option and "falling off the wagon" should truly not happen. Eating crappy, garbage foods that ultimately does more harm than good is not an option. For example, if you asked a hard core vegetarian to a steak restaurant they would say..."I don't eat meat"...not an option. If you asked a non-smoker to come out for a smoke with you, they would say, "No thanks. I don't smoke"...not an option.

People would never in their wildest dreams ask me to hit the local McDonald's with them. They just know that no matter how busy, or how hungry I am, not an option.

What are the foods that you need to make "not an option"? White bread? Fast food? Artificial sweeteners? Soda? There are plenty of foods that could never be eaten again for the rest of your life and you would be perfectly fine. Actually, you would be more than fine, There are foods that ARE still an option. If I go to a party and there is a dessert I want to try, I go for it. I don't normally eat the whole thing, but I don't deprive myself. I have it, and then move on with my healthy life. No big deal. Decide today which foods for you are not an option and then make a firm decision that your life will be so much better without them

Bodies were designed to accept and function best on natural ingredients. All aspects of humans' lives and all the systems of human bodies are impacted positively or negatively by what is ingested. Pesticides and chemicals were not meant for human consumption. Turkeys are a simple example of foods impacted by processing. We believe that the meat from these birds is good for us.

After all, turkey is the prime centerpiece on many a holiday table. Yet, the feet of many turkeys never touch the ground. They are housed in large overcrowded coops and walk on wire mesh. They are fed chemically enhanced seeds which accelerate growth. Their meat is generally white, which means little, if any, nutrients have been allowed to circulate through their bodies. Finally, before they are slaughtered, they are forced to down brine . . . a salty soup. Finally, after being slaughtered, the bodies are dipped in acid to help wash away the feathers. Sounds delicious, huh?

If there is to be a bottom line in the discussion of processed food vs. natural foods, it is that processed foods have far more bad going for them than good. Yes, I realize that finances are always a factor when it comes to eating. Not everyone can afford to eat the best foods. The best I can recommend to many of you is to wash your fruits and vegetables, but to try to eat organic foods whenever possible.

And, here's another little fact that may surprise many of you: we would be better off by eating more than five servings of fruit and vegetables per day. We should consume less than 30 grams of processed meat daily. In addition, and these are no-brainers, smoking and consumption of alcohol should be reduced to nothing . . . or, at least next to nothing. Finally, exercising 150 minutes each week is the very least you can do for your body in terms of maintaining great muscle tone and cardiovascular function.

Vitamin D is your friend. No matter where you live, you have to go out into the sun and vitamin D will help ward off the sun's harmful effects. Vitamin D can also help ward off serious diseases. And, yes, it also functions as a natural steroid for your body.

Lastly, and I realize this may be difficult for many to accept, but foods high in sugar are to be avoided. That's right, candy lovers, foods with high concentrations of processed sugars should be eaten minimally, at best. They taste great, but they're really not good for you. On a lighter note, a few beers, a bit of cake or even a carbonated drink in the course of a week won't hurt you. Remember here, however, less is more!

My recommendation here is to spend a little time on the internet to learn about proper nutrition. You just may be surprised the harm some foods may do, and pleasantly surprised to learn just how easy it is to do right by your body.

Quote from this chapter

Bodies were designed to accept and function best on natural ingredients. All aspects of humans' lives and all the systems of human bodies are impacted positively or negatively by what is ingested. Pesticides and chemicals were not meant for human consumption.

Decide today which foods for you are not an option and then make a firm decision that your life will be so much better without them

**"I took the only route that made sense,
I began to get healthy. I changed everything
about me. This included: my diet, my sleep
habits, my drinking, my exercise regimen,
and my outlook on life."**

CHAPTER 3

LIVING THE DREAM

I'm still learning more about life and about myself each and every day

The current pop phrase to indicate that life isn't going all that well for an individual is "living the dream." You may have heard it.

"How's it going, Fred?"

"Oh, I'm just living the dream."

What the respondent is actually saying in this case is, "Nothing has changed. I'm in a rut. Life is bleak. I'm not happy, and I doubt if I ever will be!"

These days when I'm asked how I'm doing, I can honestly reply that I'm living the dream . . . in the positive sense. I see, hear, taste, smell, and touch the wonder in everything . . . and I marvel at it . . . I relish it . . . and I thrive. Life isn't just beautiful; it's grand!

My brother is never quite happy. He just turned 90 years old, and is a chronic complainer. Wherever he goes, he thinks, "they're all kids." When he goes to where older people are (although, not many are older) he complains, "they're all old." He has outlived most of his friends, but he is happy to be alive. And, truly, he looks forward to a longer life. Interestingly, he recently survived bypass surgery. That was four months ago. Now, he's out playing golf three times a week! That's made him happy again. How did he survive that procedure at age 90? He was in excellent shape. Before his surgery, he would walk the 18 holes of golf every time he played. He refused to ride in the cart. On top of that, most evenings he searched out places where he could dance the night away. He hardly ever relaxed. He was always on the go. Always keeping his mind and body active.

We constantly marvel at seniors doing things that are incredible for as old as they are. "Oh, look, that lady is 80 and she's getting a Ph.d." "My word, that 90-year old is going sky diving . . . again." "Oh, my, Helen is 89 and she has a date with a man half her age.   Can you believe it?"

Maybe we should stop being amazed when folks just plain exercise their desire to do what they want to do while they are alive. If they have the talent to achieve an advanced degree, I say, "More power to 'em!" If they want to jump out of a perfectly good aircraft, I say, "Right on, buddy, go for it!"

I would be kidding myself if I thought I was the same man I was forty, let alone sixty years ago! I'm not. I'm different. I certainly have changed. I'm not necessarily less of a person, but I am a different me. You might ask, "Okay, Jack, just how are you different?" Well, I'm not necessarily wealthy in the monetary sense of the word. That fact hasn't changed perceptibly over the decades. I am, however, wealthy in terms of having true friends and dedicated family members. Amazingly, the numbers of both individuals in both groups don't appear to be diminishing; they're growing! Also, and this is important, I'm wealthy in terms of the practical wisdom I have accrued. Moreover, I'm wealthy in terms of developing and keeping a positive outlook on life

Is my outlook keeping me from aging? One has only to gaze upon my snow-capped white head to know that certainly is not true. I am growing older chronologically, but I am staying young and vital mentally, socially and spiritually. If this is true, and I believe it is, I am managing to greatly slow my aging processes because of how I embrace life. To me, life is a gift . . . or better yet, a series of gifts, and they come in the form of days. Each day is a treasure, worth its weight in gold, depending on how I use it.

Am I the great guru on aging? Far from it! You must bear in mind that I didn't see the light until I was 84, and I was a disastrous 84 at that! The good news is that I'm still alive, and I'm still learning more about life, and about myself, each and every day. In terms of the wealth I am accruing, my bank account is still very much open. I'm adding to the credit column all the time. I have become the First National Bank of Daly, and business is thriving!

Do you remember the last words spoken by Vito Corelone in the book, The Godfather. He said, "Life is beautiful." What a shame that those were his last words. It's too bad that he didn't figure that out a couple of years before he took his last breath. Who knows what kind of fun and frivolity ol' Vito could have had in his golden years!

Speaking of movies, several years ago, Walter Matheau and Jack Lemmon starred in "Grumpy Old Men". The movie was so brilliant, that the studio saw the wisdom of producing a sequel, "Grumpier Old Men". The movie focuses on two codgers who have known each other since childhood. Through time, they become set in their ways; irritated with the world, and distant from one another. The only one thing can save the day and the relationship of these curmudgeons is, of course, love. Ah, and how easy it is to soften a man's disposition when their love interests are Sophia Lauren and Ann-Margaret! It is important to note that Walter and Jack, no matter how bitter they were toward one another, managed to stay healthy through all of those years.

Health and love, what an amazing combination! It's right up there with peaches and cream and Ozzie and Harriet. I am certain that most everyone will agree, if you have your health you are truly alive. And, if you are truly alive, you are in love with the world. And, if you are in love with the world, perhaps the world will come around to loving you. And, if the world loves you, it isn't inconceivable for one individual to become your prime squeeze.

Now, back to getting better.

As I mentioned earlier, I was living, barely living, and labouring under the gross misconception that I was Grade A, U.S. Prime. The truth was that I was anything but. Death was at my door, and he wasn't just knocking, he was pounding to get inside! I took the only route that made sense, I began to get healthy. I changed everything about me. This included: my diet, my sleep habits, my drinking, my exercise regimen, and my outlook on life. Some six months later, the new and improved me is prowling the world with a wonderfully optimistic attitude. Not only do I view life more positively, I'm really, truly enjoying it! My walks are taking me by gardens and the New Hampshire seacoast. The smells and the sights are absolutely breath-taking. I hear kids playing outside my door, and music (not necessarily my particular favorites) being played from car radios. And I smile. I have been given a second chance at life and this time I'm really living it!
"

Quotes from this chapter

"And I smile. I have been given a second chance at life, and this time I'm really living it!"

"I am certain that most everyone will agree, if you have your health, you are truly alive. And, if you are truly alive, you are in love with the world. And, if you are in love with the world, perhaps the world will come around to loving you."

"The good news is that I'm still alive, and I'm still learning more about life, and about myself, each and every day."

**Always remember to forget the
troubles that pass your way;
BUT NEVER forget the blessings
that come each day**

GREAT TRUTHS THAT
ADULTS HAVE LEARNED:

1) Raising teenagers is like nailing jelly to a tree.
2) Wrinkles don't hurt.
3) Families are like fudge...mostly sweet, with a few nuts
4) Today's mighty oak is just yesterday's nut that held its ground.
5) Laughing is good exercise. It's like jogging on the inside.
6) Middle age is when you choose your cereal for the fiber, not the toy.

GREAT TRUTHS
ABOUT GROWING OLD

1) Growing old is mandatory; growing up is optional..
2) Forget the health food. I need all the preservatives I can get.
3) When you fall down, you wonder what else you can do while you're down there.
4) You're getting old when you get the same sensation from a rocking chair that you once got from a roller coaster.
5) It's frustrating when you know all the answers but nobody bothers to ask you the questions.
6) Time may be a great healer, but it's a lousy beautician
7) Wisdom comes with age, but sometimes age comes alone.

THE SENILITY PRAYER:
God, grant me the senility to forget the people I never liked anyway, the good fortune to run into those that I do, and the eyesight to tell the difference.

"I'm not fishing, I'm reading"

A couple goes on vacation to a fishing resort in northern Minnesota. The husband likes to fish at the crack of dawn. The wife likes to read. One morning the husband returns after several hours of fishing and decides to take a nap. She motors out a short distance, anchors, and continues to read her book. Along comes a game warden in his boat. He pulls up alongside the woman and says, "Good morning Ma'am. What are you doing?" Reading a book," she replies — thinking, "Isn't that > obvious?" "You're in a restricted fishing area," he informs her. "I'm sorry officer, but I'm not fishing, I'm reading" "Yes, but you have all the equipment. For all I know you could start at any moment. I'll have to take you in and write you up." "If you do that, I'll have to charge you with sexual assault," says the woman. "But I haven't even touched you," says the game warden. "That's true, but you have all the equipment. For all I know you could start at any moment." "Have a nice day ma'am", and he left. MORAL: Never argue with a woman who reads; it's likely she also thinks

Three men married wives from different countries

The first man married a woman from China.
He told her that she was to do their dishes and house cleaning. It took a couple of days, but on the third day, he came home to see a clean house and dishes washed and put away. The second man married a woman from Italy. He gave his wife orders that she was to do all the cleaning, dishes and the cooking. The first day he didn't see any results, but the next day he saw it was better. By the third day, he saw his house was clean, the dishes were done and there was a huge dinner on the table The third man married a girl from America He ordered her to keep the house cleaned, dishes washed, lawn mowed, laundry washed, and hot meals on the table for every meal. He said the first day he didn't see anything, the second day he didn't see anything but by the third day, some of the swelling had gone down and he could see a little out of his left eye, and his arm was healed enough that he could fix himself a sandwich and load the dishwasher. "Isn't it amazing? We, each of us, receive the gift of a new day, each and every day of out lives. What we do with that gift is the choice that really matters."

Silver in the Hair. Gold in the Teeth. Stones in the Kidneys. Sugar in the Blood. Lead in the Feet. Iron in the Arteries. And an inexhaustible supply of Natural Gas We never thought we'd accumulate such wealth.

How do you stay looking so young?

One day, while strolling down the boardwalk, John bumped into an old friend of his, Rob, from high school. "You look great John, how do you stay looking so young? Why you must be 60 already but you don't look a day over 40!" Rob exclaimed. "I feel like I'm 40 too!" replied John. "That's incredible" exclaimed Rob, "Does it run in the family? How old was your dad when he passed?" "Did I say he was dead?" asked John. "He's 81 and is more active then ever. He just joined the neighborhood basketball team!" responded John. "Whoa! Well how old was your Grandfather when he died?" "Did I say he died" asked John. Rob was amazed. "He just had his 105th birthday and plays golf and goes swimming each day! He's actually getting married this week!" "Getting married?!" Rob asked. If he's 105, why on earth does he want to get married?! John looked at Rob and replied, "Did I say he wanted to?"

I have anticipated that the results of aging will occur, and I'm moving on with my life

CHAPTER 4
AGING GRACEFULLY

I believe that successful aging must include finding and accomplishing meaningful things.

. To age gracefully does not mean to give in and give up. Changes to the body are inevitable. We should expect those changes. Our health will inevitably plateau downward. We will become more vulnerable to illness and injury. Those are facts. Deal with them! You'll hear many old timers complaining that they've lost their teeth, their hearing, their eyesight, and, finally, "you-know-what." With all of the problems existing in the world, if the most you have to get you down is that you can't get it up . . . you, my friend, are doing well!

Those of us who live in New England have the occasion to watch maple trees turn into maple shoots. They, in turn, become saplings. In time, those saplings become full-fledged shade trees. Those trees lose branches in storms and are subject to disease or preying insects. The point is that those magnificent old trees we love to photograph in the fall bear almost no resemblance to the young saplings they once were. I'm not certain of this, but I don't believe that those great maples rue the day that they stopped looking like saplings and became majestic and stately.

I have accepted the inevitable changes of aging. I see

changes almost daily, but I don't see each as a crisis. I have anticipated that the results of aging will occur, and I'm moving on with my life. I'm getting older, but I'm working at being productive. I'm not 95 yet, but I hope that if I reach that plateau I still see life as a marvel. I would hope that I can continue to be the type of person other people want to be around. I would hope that I can still care for myself and still have ideas others might consider to be profound. In other words, I am going to strive to age gracefully. I have this one body and one mind. If I work at it daily, I should be able to keep body and soul together for some years to come. Moreover, I hope to appreciate the wonders of life until my life leaves me. At present, I maintain my own apartment and drive my own car. I'm looking forward to my next business venture, and I know the names of just about everybody I work out with in the gym. I'm working at staying vital. I strive to be alive. I find joy in the smiles of others. I may not be the happiest camper in the forest, but at least I'm still camping!

The older you become, the greater the chances that you have survived threats to your physical and psychological integrity. You have lost family and friends. Through good luck or good genes, or both, some older people have dodged fatal accidents and disease. You have made good decisions about living. You are strong and can hope to live a long, productive life. Most people think that is a benefit. I know I do.

As I age, I continually hear folks saying things such as, "My memory is going." I'm slowing down." "I'm constantly going to wakes and funerals. What's the point?" You have to, and this is a must, have important things before you to accomplish. You need to be positive about the people and events in your life. You need to have a purposeful retirement. You need to maintain your personal health and mental wellbeing. And, under no circumstances, should you give in to those negative anchors which can only drag you down.

Many of us know someone who has lost a husband or a wife, someone they have been with for many years. Until the time of their death the mate, the soul mate, was that individual's heart and inspiration. Sadly, a number of those people who have suffered that loss see no reason to continue to live and pass away in a very short time after their loss. The tragedy is that the survivor could find no reason to go on with life. Essentially, when the spouse cashed in his chips, so did the survivor.

It is tough to continue to go on in life, but I believe we must persevere. I believe that each of us should make every effort to acquire all that life has to offer for as long as we can. We didn't choose to be born, but we were given the gift of life. How sad, I believe, it is to say, "I don't like this hand. Deal me out!"

I feel each of us has some regrets. Perhaps we have wasted time; spent more time with the family; developed a talent or achieved a particular goal. I try not to rationalize my shortcomings, but I have come to realize that my imperfections only indicate that I am human. I do strive each day to be better, and I only hope that the gift of my life has true meaning to others.

Is "aging joyfully" an oxymoron? It could be but I really don't think so. Certainly, living is a death-defying feat, and growing older is a major accomplishment. Some folks believe that because their hearts still beat and they have all of the other vital signs in working order that they are living. Well, technically, they are correct. But are they really living in the sense that they are leading useful, vital lives? Ah, that point is highly debatable.

If you are really living, you see the value of your life. You appreciate those around you, even if you may have differences of opinions. You see yourself as a brick in the wall in your community . . . you value yourself, your place in your family, your place in social and religious organizations. You recognize the accomplishments of others throughout history, and you recognize your own accomplishments. You're not willing to throw in the towel as you tack on the birthdays, You see yourself as someone knowledgeable in a field and willing to share your expertise or be an example to those who aspire to follow in your footsteps.

Sir Michael Caine is aging gracefully and productively. He has appeared in over 115 films and shows no signs of stopping any time soon. Caine was born in 1933 and served with the British army in Korea. He swears he knew he was going to die in battle, but if he were to live he would really live every moment for the rest of his life. Caine took up acting while in his 20's and knew he had found his life's calling. "Be like a duck," said Caine. "Calm on the surface, but paddling like the dickens underneath." He also recognized that many actors have their moments in the sun and bow out the public eye. He was not about to let that happen. He worked to find roles that would accommodate his persona throughout the various stages of this life. From the dashing young lieutenant in Zulu in 1964 to the aging, but devoted butler in The Dark Knight Rises in 2012, Sir Michael Caine continues to be a vital force on stage and screen. On aging, Caine said, "I think life has got to develop as you get older, and I don't want to be wandering along doing the same old thing. I want more out of life."

Allow me to pause and provide my definition of "aging gracefully." First of all, what it is not is aging elegantly. I have nothing against the Queen of England, but she might be considered to be one who is aging elegantly. Every hair is in place, and her heart rate probably never exceeds 30 beats per minute. Ronald Reagan might be considered one who aged gracefully. If you remember, in his 80's, long after he had left the White House, he still managed to stay vital at the Reagan ranch by chopping wood and doing other ranch chores. Now, he was a man who could stay on task!

I believe that successful aging must include finding and accomplishing meaningful things. Those folks who while away their hours feeding the pigeons or playing checkers are doing just that . . . whiling away their hours. The people I know who are aging well aren't thinking about getting older; they're thinking about doing. They're thinking about visiting someone in need. They're thinking about the next employment project they can initiate. They're thinking about finding that rattle under the trunk of the car and fixing it. They're thinking about the dinner they are about to make for the company the're inviting over on Friday night. They are exercising, staying sharp intellectually, and finding every reason to be happy. What they are not doing is focusing on their aches and pains. They are not focusing on negative factors over which they have no control. They are living life, and they are a pleasure to be with

Quotes from this chapter

"I have accepted the inevitable changes of aging. I see changes almost daily, but I don't see each as a crisis. I have anticipated that the results of aging will occur, and I'm moving on with my life."

"It is tough to continue to go on in life, but I believe we must persevere. I believe that each of us should make every effort to acquire all that life has to offer for as long as we can."

Softly stroking face with both hands

A woman went up up the bar in a quiet rural pub. She gestured alluringly to the bartender who approached her immediately She seductively signaled that he should bring his face closer to hers. As he did, she gently caressed his full beard. "Are you the manager?" she asked, softly stroking his face with both hands. "Actually, no," he replied "Can you get him for me?" I need to speak to him," she said, running her hands beyond his beard and into his hair. "I'm afraid I can't," breathed the bartender.."is there anything I can do." "Yes, I need you to give him a message," she continued, running her forefinger across the bartender's lip and slyly popping a couple of her fingers into his mouth and allowing him to suck them gently. "What should I tell him?" the bartender managed to say. "Tell him," she whispered. "there's no toilet paper, hand soap, or paper towels in the ladies room."

Aerobics class for seniors

I feel like my body has gotten totally out of shape, I got my doctor's permission to join a fitness club and start exercising. I decided to take an aerobics class for seniors. I bent, twisted, gyrated, jumped up and down, and perspired for an hour. But, by the time I got my leotards on the class was over.

CHAPTER 5

MAKE EACH MOMENT COUNT

ENJOY THE GIFT OF A NEW DAY

"Each day is a gift. I'll focus on the new day and all of the happy memories I've stored away"

Isn't it amazing? We, each of us, receive the gift of a new day, each and every day of out lives. What we do with that gift is the choice that really matters. Each of us knows the expression, "wasting time." If each of us was given a lifetime of 100 years, just how much of that would be wasted on complaining . . . wasted on gossiping . . . wasted not utilizing our talents . . . wasted giving into our addictions . . . wasted on not making the world a better place? Sadly, the answer to that question could probably be stated in decades. And, since most of us won't live to be one hundred years-old, the percentage of wasted time in our lives will be that much greater.

Sickness and operations are major concerns for the elderly. I knew I was beginning to age when my body parts began to go south. First, it was my teeth. The next was my hearing. The third was my "you-know-what," (but more about that later). The fourth was my heart, which necessitated in my need for a triple-bypass operation. The next thing to go will, most likely, be me.

Call it what you will . . good luck, good friends, or an angel on my shoulder . . .I survived a life-threatening disease that required me to lug an oxygen tank behind me. Man, talk about a wake-up call! I came to the immediate realization that I needed a solution to live a full life and be sickness-free. Now, some people might turn to God for their solutions; I turned to

WELLNESS for mine. And what is wellness? Wellness is the quality or state of being in good health that actively seeks to perpetuate all that is positive. Much as negative forces in a person's lifestyle causes that individual to spiral downward, wellness, and all that is positive, causes that individual to spiral upward (metaphorically speaking, of course).

It was so simple, yet, so profound. I became an instant convert to the Church of Wellness. I immediately joined an exercise facility and began to cut down drastically on my food and alcohol intake. I began to stay away from fatty foods and I started walking. SHAZAM! The magic worked. Within a month I wasn't coughing and wheezing. I didn't need oxygen, and I ceased to think of doctors and nurses as my new BFF's! In a nutshell, I felt great..

Good friends tell the truth. As I mentioned earlier, one of my best friends told me I still had a long life ahead of me, if I would only take better care of my body. I did, and I'm alive to tell you about it. That being said, allow me to tell you about "J.B."

Joe "J.B." Butler is a good friend of mine. He has a vast amount of stories of his time aboard the USS Izard, a Fletcher-class destroyer, lovingly called a "tin can" during World War II. The Izard didn't receive a great deal of notoriety, but it usually held the point position when Butler's squadron would go into battle. "I know how precious life is," he would say, "I saw a lot of good men, many of them my buddies, lose their lives in bitter battles out there on the high seas. As a gunnery mate, J.B had fought in every battle in the Pacific Theater of Operations except one. By war's end, J.B. had lost 60% of his hearing. In addition, his once trim physique and perfect health had begun to sag. It became obvious to many that he wasn't the man he was just a short while ago. A good friend of his suggested that he become acquainted with "chair exercises" promoted by the Royal Canadian Mounted Police. At first, he doubted that these simple exercises could be effective. "How could they be," he chuckled. "You would just sit there and move about. I thought it was a joke, but I tried it." J.B. is now

90 and a daily practitioner of that short regimen . By the way, he looks great!

Thanks to my own good friend, and my wellness and exercise program, I now feel FANTASTIC! I never would have believed that regaining good health could be this easy. Can something as simple as a few exercises, walking and a diet change make a difference? I'm living proof that it can!

Since I had my scare (which sounds a great deal like "boo," but felt more like BBBBOOOO!!! to the 10th power), I have been grateful each and every day for the gift of a new day. Knowing how self-destructive and self-centered I was, I am now so very concerned that I try to do right by the world.

Dear Reader, I'm really making an effort to have you walk a mile in my moccasins. Moreover, I'm attempting to have you not walk in them. I'm being very forthright here; I'm telling you that I nearly died through no fault but my own. I'm telling you, I was holding on by my fingernails. The future didn't just look bleak; it looked nonexistent. Somehow, I was allowed a second chance. I was offered a second shot at life, and I'm trying to make each moment count. I'm trying to make memories, and I'm trying to savor all of them.

My advice to you is to begin each day as though you're opening that special gift at Christmas. You remember that gift . . . the one you always wanted . . . the one you were going to take very good care of and never, ever lend to anybody else. And, then you got it! You took it in your hands, so careful not to break it as you tore the paper and bow from the box. Your eyes went wide. Your mouth formed a perfect O, and you had to force yourself to breathe. Well, today you received that very special gift, yet again. With luck, you'll receive it again tomorrow . . . and the day after that . . . and the day after that. Those gifts won't go on forever. You have to make some choices . . . wise, adult choices. Will you squander them away, or will you do something magnificent?

It took some time for Bill Murray's character in the movie Groundhog Day to understand the concept of life as daily gift. Thankfully, he did. He got it, and he became a better man because he did.

Okay, here comes the tough love. No one is going to take you by the hand to help you along through this journey of life. That's your job. No one is going to stick a star on your forehead or pat you on the back each time you do the right thing. Conversely, not many folks are going to be kind enough to let you know when you're not doing so well either. Consider this book to be your wake-up call. Consider me to be your personal Dalai Lama and these few words to be the gospel of wellness. This is your one chance at life. Remember that slogan for the U.S. Army, "Be all that you can be?" Do you? Well, good.   NOW, DO IT!

I already decided to love it. It's a decision I make every day when I wake up

The 92-year old lady was petite, well-poised and proud. She was fully dressed each morning by eight o'clock. Her hair was fashionably coiffed, and her make-up was applied with precision care, even though she was legally blind.

Her husband of 70 years recently passed away, so she made the necessary arrangements to move into a nursing home. On her arrival, she had to wait several hours while her room was being prepped. When she was told her room was ready, she accompanied the attendant to the elevator. On the way, the attendant described her tiny new quarters.

I love it," squealed the woman.

"But, how can you love it," asked the attendant." You haven't even seen it."

"I love it," stated the woman, "because I made up my mind to do so. Happiness is something you decide on ahead of time. Whether I like my room or not doesn't depend on how the furniture is arranged. It is how I arrange my mind. I already decided to love it. It's a decision I make every day when I wake up. I have a choice. I can spend the day in bed with the parts of my body that no longer work, or I can get out of bed and be thankful for the ones that do. Each day is a gift. And, as long as my eyes are open, I'll focus on the new day and all of the happy memories I've stored away . . . just for this time in my new life."

Health and Wellness

Health is a dynamic process because it is always changing. We all have times of good health, times of sickness, and maybe even times of serious illness. As our lifestyles change, so does our level of health. Those of us who participate in regular physical activity do so partly to improve the current and future level of our health. We strive toward an optimal state of well-being. As our lifestyle improves, our health also improves and we experience less disease and sickness. When most people are asked what it means to be healthy they normally respond with the four components of fitness mentioned earlier (cardiorespiratory ability, muscular ability, flexibility, and body composition). Although these components are a critical part of being healthy, they are not the only contributing factors. Physical health is only one aspect of our overall health

INNOCENCE IS PRICELESS

One Sunday morning, the pastor noticed little Alex standing in the foyer of the church staring up at a large plaque. It was covered with names and small American flags mounted on both sides of it. The six-year old had been staring at the plaque for some time, so the pastor walked up, stood beside the little boy, and said quietly, "Good morning Alex."

"Good morning Pastor," he replied, still focused on the plaque. "Pastor, what is this?"

The pastor said, "Well son, it's a memorial to all the young men and women who died in the service."

Soberly, they just stood together, staring at the large plaque.

Finally, little Alex's voice, barely audible and trembling with fear asked, "Which service, the 8:30 or the 10:30?"

"I certainly hope it isn't loaded!"

I was once asked by a lady visiting if I had a gun in the house. I said I did. She said 'Well I certainly hope it isn't loaded!' To which I said, of course it is loaded, can't work without bullets!' She then asked, 'Are you that afraid of someone evil coming into your house?' My reply was, 'No not at all. I am not afraid of the house catching fire either, but I have fire extinguishers around, and they are all loaded too.' To which I'll add, having a gun in the house that isn't loaded is like having a car in the garage without gas in the tank

**While I'm meeting, greeting and working out,
I am releasing endorphins into my body."**

CHAPTER 6

WORKING OUT

Smiling while you sweat . . . what a concept! Life is truly beautiful, isn't it

I have met so many wonderful people at the exercise facility I recently joined. Many of them have become great acquaintances, and a few have become really wonderful friends. One element of being a friend or acquaintance is having something in common with the other person. I can't think of a better way to develop a relationship based on a commonality than to share a regular workout experience. Both of you are there to work at getting back in shape, and both of you may be of a similar age. Obviously, you both live in the same community, and both of you may hurt if you are both mutually out of shape.

And, there is the encouragement factor. One person working out alone just may become discouraged. Becoming discouraged is easy enough to do. The lone person hurts, and begins to question just why he or she ever considered joining that stupid gym anyway. What a dumb idea! But, add another hurting rookie to the mix, and you have a great recipe. You begin to laugh at pain. You truly look forward to seeing that other individual on the treadmill next to yours. You begin to see improvement in the person's overall appearance. You may even tell them so, and you'll be surprised when they tell you the same thing. Amazingly, both of you are telling the truth.! Who would ever believe that the foundation of a great relationship could be based on sweat?

Smiling while you sweat . . . what a concept! Life is truly beautiful, isn't it?

Speaking of smiling, I'm doing a lot of that lately. No, I'm really not getting completely silly in my old age; I smile because I have an overall sense of joy and wellbeing. I have acquired that feeling because I am working out. When I work out, I continue to meet and greet people. While I'm meeting, greeting and working out, I am releasing endorphins into my body. Those little devils help to drive up my natural sense of euphoria, and that euphoric feeling doesn't slam shut when the workout session is over . . . not by a long shot. They are with me for quite a while, and I only add to them when I return to the gym the next day. It is as though I am making unlimited withdrawals from my bank, and my bank account keeps on growing! Amazing, huh?

Oh, by the way, those endorphins help to make me really nice to be around. Believe it or not, this 84-year old still has sex appeal. You wouldn't believe how many times I have been flirted with while I work up a sweat. The return to the gym has done wonderful things for my sex life, but more about that later.

By making friends at the gym, we also encourage one another to eat, drink and live in a healthy manner.

Since you've both bought a ticket on this same life trip, you may as well share the experience. How wonderful it is to know that you are motivating someone who is also motivating you.

I recently met an elderly lady while shopping. We were both searching out juices, and we struck up a conversation. I soon found out that she is a year younger than I. I also found out that she felt miserable. Her legs ached. Her back ached. She had problems sleeping, and she didn't look forward to eating. I was almost embarrassed to tell her just how great I felt, but I did. I told her about my gym experience. I told her that I was an apostle of wellness, and that I would welcome her to the gym anytime she chose to attend. Quite honestly, I didn't think she was taking me seriously. Well, she did! She has been a regular now for several weeks, and I have to tell you that there is a certain aura about her . . . I mean she is glowing with health. She has thanked me several times for directing her to the on-ramp of health and happiness. For my part, I'm just gratified to learn that she is once again enjoying life.

She and I have become good friends, or maybe the best of acquaintances. We share a smile and an occasional joke. We encourage each other. We inspire each other. We sweat.

C'mon, let's hear it! Yeah, life!

Some of us really have no friends, and that's a true pity. Some of us think we have friends, but they are really acquaintances. It is important that we understand the difference between a friend and an acquaintance. A friend will give you the shirt off of his back. An acquaintance will give you the shirt off of his back, but he'll want a receipt!

Please don't misunderstand me, acquaintances are great to have. They're great to have when you're trying to get up a poker game. Hey, they may even bring the beer! They may even share their middle names, but acquaintances just seem to drift in and out of our lives without really being a meaningful part of it. Sometimes, we may put too much stock in a relationship with an acquaintance, and feel angry or sad when it comes to an end. Some of us wear our hearts on our sleeves; some are there just to take us to the cleaners

I've been taken. I suppose all of us have. The experience is humiliating, but the really good news is that most of us don't give up on all others. We're willing to take that risk of friendship again and again.

Quote from this chapter

"You truly look forward to seeing that other individual on the treadmill next to yours. You begin to see improvement in the person's overall appearance. You may even tell them so, and you'll be surprised when they tell you the same thing."

Here is what a few famous people had to offer:

A friend is one of the nicest things you can have, and one of the best things you can be. Douglas Pagels

The antidote for fifty enemies is one friend. Aristotle

A good friend is cheaper than therapy. Author Unknown

The most I can do for my friend is simply to be his friend.
 Henry David Thoreau

The most beautiful discovery true friends make is that they can grow separately without growing apart.
Elisabeth Foley

A friend is the one who comes in when the whole world goes out. Grace Pulpit

The language of friendship is not words, but meanings.
Henry David Thoreau

A true friend reaches for your hand and touches your heart.
Attributed to Heather Pryor.

About Best Friends...

Best friends are people who make your problems their problems, just so you don't have to go through them alone

Here's to the nights that turned into morning with the friends that turned into family

There is nothing better than a friend, unless it is a friend with chocolate.

"I can't think of your name"

Two elderly ladies had been best of friends for decades. Over the years, they shared all kinds of activities and adventures. Of late, however, their activities had been limited to meeting a few times a week to play cards. One day, they were playing when one looked at the other and said, "Now don't get mad . . . I know we've been friends for years, but I can't think of your name. I've thought and thought, but I can't remember it. Please tell me what your name is." Her friend glared at her for at least three minutes. Finally, she said, "How soon do you need to know?"

At the Salon

I overheard the receptionist admit to another customer, "I haven't taken my vitamins today. I'm walking around unprotected." The customer commiserated with her, but then added, "I haven't taken my Prozac today—everyone's walking around unprotected."

Oh, the pity of old age.

When I went to lunch today, I noticed an old man sitting on a park bench sobbing his eyes out. I stopped and asked him what was wrong. He said, "I have a 22 year old wife at home. She rubs my back every morning and then gets up and makes me pancakes, sausage, fresh fruit and freshly ground coffee."

I said, "Well, then why are you crying?"

He said, "She makes me homemade soup for lunch and my favorite brownies, cleans the house and then watches sports TV with me for the rest of the afternoon."

I said, "Well, why are you crying?"

He said, "For dinner she makes me a gourmet meal with wine and my favorite dessert and then makes love with me until the wee hours."

I said, "Well, why in the world would you be crying?"

He said, "I can't remember where I live!"

"It's okay to have achy muscles. If you ache, it means you're still alive enough to know that you haven't used, or properly used, your muscles in some time.

CHAPTER 7

ADVENTURE OF HARD EXERCISE

ALL THOSE ACHES AND PAINS?

You may even find yourself actually smiling at all of those miniscule aches and pains

The good news is that those aches are temporary. You can muzzle that screaming by simply continuing to work out and taking proper care of your body before and after each workout session. The big ticket here is not to rationalize. Let me say that again . . . DON'T RATIONALIZE! Because you exercised on Monday doesn't mean that you also covered Tuesday through Sunday. Because your legs ache doesn't give you a free pass until they stop aching. For you sports fans, you just may understand this better by believing that you have made your favorite pro team, and that you are in pre-season training for the big game. And, the big game is THE REST OF YOUR LIFE!

You probably know all of the locker room clichés, but in case you don't here are a few: When the going gets rough, the rough get going! Stick to a task, 'til it sticks to you! It's not the size of the dog in the fight; it's the amount of fight in the dog!

Those simple clichés are meant to bolster and to challenge. I don't know who came up with them, but they wouldn't have been said at all if someone didn't need to hear them. That means, basically, that you are not the first person who needs to shape up. You are not the first person who is facing a death sentence if you don't. You are not the first person who wants to quit and bow out of the race, but you're reading this book. You're pondering the words you are reading. You're imagining yourself in better shape, and you're imagining yourself enjoying a long, fruitful life. Well, congratulations, you have just taken the first step on your journey of one thousand miles.

Okay, let me play psychic here. You've just had your first thought. It was good. It came from that cheerful little voice in your right ear. Right behind, a loud, nasty voice called out in your left year. It said, "Yeah, but what am I going to get with all those aches and pains? Is it really worth the trouble?"

The answer is that you are going to achieve an amazing sense of satisfaction. All of those endorphins that you have activated are going to have a ball coursing through your revitalized body. You may even find yourself actually smiling at all of those miniscule aches and pains. You may even hear the music from Rocky blasting into your brain as you are toweling down after your shower. You will strut to the mirror, snarl and say, "You are a lean, mean, fighting machine!" Okay, okay, maybe I got a little ahead of myself there. The good news is that when the same activity is repeated continually, the muscle will respond to it. You are creating a positive muscle memory, and you will have no soreness, or, at least less soreness. What you are doing in each work out is to strengthen your muscles and your connective tissue.

Here's some more good news. That osteoarthritis you have been developing as you have been aging will start to dissipate with each warm-up and workout session. And, ladies and gentlemen, I am here to tell you that nothing, but nothing, feels better than to be pain free. I'm not promising miracles here, but with each workout session you just may find your accumulated aches and pains gradually diminishing to the point of nothingness. Is that a smile I see on your face? I believe it is. You want to be pain-free, don't you? You want a longer life, don't you? You want to be productive and in better shape? Yeah, you bet you do!

I'm not asking you to send your hard-earned dollars in for some gizmo that will melt the pounds away. I'm simply saying that you have it within yourselves to healthier and happier, and happier because you will be healthier.

Here's your homework . . . Don't give up! You can do it!

I believe that people generally know what is good for them. They know that reading improves the mind. They know that drinking excessive alcoholic beverages can ruin the liver. They know that eight hours of sleep a night is ideal, and they know that regular workouts improve muscle tone, breathing, and cardiovascular function. Does that stop people from not reading, drinking too much, sleeping very little and not being physically fit? Nope. People are humans, and humans are prone to rationalize and take the easy way out. And, yes, for the record . . . I'm human, too!

As I've mentioned, I somehow managed to achieve 84 years on this planet, but I was in lousy condition. I was very close to the register in the eternal check-out line, but I made a conscious effort to really clean up my act and live properly.

Prior to THE BIG SCARE, my concept of exercise was tossing and turning at night. I wasn't doing much of anything to keep body and soul together. If my body had been a car, it would have been junked years ago. But, THE BIG SCARE is a giant bucket of cold water thrown in my face. I could have gone down with no more than a whimper, or gone down swinging. I chose the latter. Looking back on the past few short months, I can't believe just how much I have achieved. Further, I can't believe that I am alive and delighted to compose this little story. You should understand that I'm not an athlete by any stretch of the imagination, but I'm not afraid to sweat a little. And, I'm certainly able to stick to a routine.

Let me try something. When one reads capital letters in bold print, one is supposed to be impressed by the importance of the print. He believes that the author is yelling directly at him. For the sake of argument, let's assume that this is true, shall we? Okay, if you want to live a long, healthy life, you need to: EXERCISE DAILY! DON'T DRINK TO EXCESS! EAT A BALANCED DIET! AND BE PRODUCTIVE!

If you're as old as I, you may remember television's Sergeant Preston of the Yukon. If you do, you'll remember that he ended each show by him patting his lead dog and saying, "Well, King, I guess this case is closed." If you take nothing from this book except what I have spelled out in Times New Roman capital letters in the paragraph above, I can honestly say, "Well, Dear Reader, I guess this case is closed.

The Chinese are wise folk, and they have a saying that is so simple and yet so profound. It should be tacked up on walls everywhere. It is "The journey of a thousand miles begins with the first step." Great, huh? You can't get anywhere if you don't take the first step . . . and the second . . . and the third. If you start moving in the right direction, you're doing something positive. If you stop, you're not.

It's okay to have achy muscles. If you ache, it means you're still alive enough to know that you haven't used, or properly used, your muscles in some time. Those muscles are yelling at you. They're cursing you, because you just woke them up. They're screaming at you, because it's easy to do nothing and turn into a bowl full of jelly. I know. I was right in the middle of that bowl!

Stick to a task till it sticks to you

Do I continue this exercising that causes me discomfort, or do I give it up and relax. What are the alternatives? If someone over 50 doesn't have any form of exercise, the body will slow down. But, If you do choose to exercise in some form you will be more physically fit and healthy which will enable you to live a better life. Stick to it and make it an essential part of your life. It could be the best decision you make at any age. Stick to a task till it sticks to you

"Never give up.

It's like breathing—once you quit, your flame dies letting total darkness extinguish every last gasp of hope. You can't do that. You must continue taking in even the shallowest of breaths, continue putting forth even the smallest of efforts to sustain your dreams. Don't ever, ever, ever give up."
☐ *Richelle E. Goodrich, Smile Anyway:*

"Don't do it!

Don't you dare think about giving up! EVERYTHING has a process. Work with the process, not against it. Move forward with purpose and never stop believing. You can do this! You know you can." ☐ *Stephanie Lahar*

"The keys to health and weight-loss: stress reduction, sleep, deep breathing, clean water, complete nutrition, sunshine, walking, stretching, meditation, love, community, laughter, dreams, perseverance, purpose, humility, action."
☐ *Bryant McGill,*

Don't trust little Old Ladies!!!

A young man shopping in a supermarket Noticed a little old lady following him around. If he stopped, she stopped. Furthermore she kept staring at him. She finally overtook him at the checkout, And she turned to him and said, "I hope I haven't made you feel ill at ease; it's just that you look so much like my late son." He answered, "That's okay." "I know it's silly, but if you'd call out

"Good bye, Mom" as I leave the store, it would make me feel so happy." She then went through the checkout, And as she was on her way out of the store, The man called out, "Good-bye, Mom." The little old lady waved, and smiled back at him pleased that he had brought a little sunshine Into someone's day, he went to pay for his groceries. "That comes to $121.85," said the clerk. "How come so much ... I only bought 5 items..." The clerk replied, "Yeah, but your Mother said you'd be paying for her things, too." Don't trust little old ladies!!!

Thinking of the hereafter

The preacher came to call the other day. He said at my age I should be thinking of the hereafter. I told him, "Oh I do it all the time. No matter where I am, in the parlor, upstairs, in the kitchen, or down in the basement, I ask myself, "Now, what am I here after?"

"If you are enjoying satisfying sex, you are certainly enjoying meaningful companionship."

CHAPTER 8

SEX, INTIMACY AND COMPANIONSHIP

I'm delighted with the healthier viewpoint on sex so many of today's middle-agers and silvers possess. No wonder people are living longer . . . those smiles aren't simply the result of jogging!

Well, here it is. You've finally reached, what you hope is, the most exciting chapter in the book. In drafting this work, I gave this particular section a great deal of thought. Of course, I could have gone with bawdy text and adult cartoons. I gave consideration to delving into the physiological, psychological and social considerations of intimate relationships, but I decided to can all of that and go with door number three. When one thinks of sex, intimacy and companionship, I believe his or her first reaction is to smile. If that is true, let's keep this simple and just maybe you can keep that smile throughout the whole chapter. Here goes . . .

When two people find that they have that certain magic, they want romance. They're not quite sure what romance is exactly, but they want it anyway. How do they achieve romance? They hold hands. They go for a walk (preferably, along the beach at sunset). They cuddle on the couch and watch television. It may be safe to assume that romance really is companionship in the sharing of quality time. Humans love quality time, and, conversely, they love companionship and romance. All of this is especially true for older folks. After all, those in the "silver set" move at a slower pace and enjoy the ability to savor quality time. I believe it is the simple things that matter most to older folks . . . a walk . . . a bike ride . . . perhaps, a camping experience. The essential item to re-member is that there is no such thing as "have to." The silvers have figured out that time shared equals greater bonding and mutual contentment.

Gentle Reader, the theme of this book is "Surviving Ill-ness." I firmly believe that the best getting better experience is done in the company of someone you absolutely want to be with until the end of time. Romance is like that perfect can-dy bar being eaten slowly in a darkened theater while your all-time favorite film is being shown. You want to make that candy last . . . and last . . . and last. You want to savor each and every bite. You want to taste that delicious treat from the opening scene to the final credits, so you do your very best to have the best possible candy/movie experience ever! Now, that is romance!

Do you remember when you were perhaps in junior high school and you first really paid attention to someone (your sex or the opposite . . . it doesn't matter). You probably didn't have a great deal of working knowledge, but you did know that you felt electrically excited. You were charged with antici-pation, but you really didn't know for what. You couldn't wait to be with that person. But, when you had the opportunity, noth-ing seemed as perfect as you had imagined it would. Luckily, time has moved on! You're better at life now. You know most of the ropes, but there just may be a little more to learn.

Having a long-term intimate relationship offers a sense of well-being. Don't let anyone kid you, there are people in the world who actually believe that they have the authority to stop seniors (and others) from participating in having sex. There are also some seniors who believe that they have reached that magic age when sex is a function that once existed but is not to be attempted any longer. My take is if you, gentle reader, stay interested in life; stay off medications; have a loving mate, then you can have good sex to the end of your life. And, if you are enjoying satisfying sex, you are certainly enjoying meaningful companionship.

Recently, I had the occasion to look at some family photos from the 60's. My relatives were old, or at least they practiced being old. I did the math, and they were in their 40's . . . but appearing as though they were in their 70's. Not only did they appear older than their ages, but they acted it! I don't know this for a fact, but I'm fairly certain that their bedrooms weren't used for anything but sleeping. So much has changed in the last four decades; I'm delighted with the healthier viewpoint on sex so many of today's middle-agers and silvers possess. No wonder people are living longer . . . those smiles aren't simply the result of jogging!

It pains me to write this, but when I was in my 40's, my first wife informed me that when she would turn 50 our sex life would cease. Sadly, what we did in the bedroom, and only in the bedroom, was infrequent at best and could have been rated PG-17. For the first twenty years of our marriage, I waited for that truly wonderful moment when we would be in sync . . . we would be in harmony . . . we could share uninhibited adult time . . . forever. It never happened!

So, I'm here to tell you, first hand, that putting a clock on sex and intimacy, or having someone dictate constraints on expressions of love is not anything that the majority of thinking, feeling adults would, or should, tolerate . . . ever!

She, my first wife, that is, wanted companionship. But is companionship better than sex? Truthfully, it is very much a part of good sex. Companionship is one of the primary building blocks of trust. Without trust, you certainly can't have good sex. I believe most of you would agree, however, that companionship without sex in an intimate, monogamous relationship, is like that candy bar without that magical chocolate center. It is just lacking.

Further, I believe that love is also essential for good sex. Sex is empty without love. Sure the physical sensations are exciting and pleasurable, but all of that dissipates quickly and leaves in its wake a sense of longing for what was missing. If loving intimacy is missing most of us feel sad, upset and cheated during, and after, the act. Without loving intimacy, it is as though we have abused our own values. When everything is in place in love-making – there is nothing that compares!

All of us, but especially those a bit older, can be sexual in order to express affection, passion, love, loyalty and appreciation of life as opposed to merely a sexual release. I acknowledge that some older folks become very limited in being able to engage in enthusiastic love-making. For them, non-sexual touch is also magical. An arm around a loved one; a small caress on the back; or a brush along the cheek with the back of hand is affirming and reassuring. Such a gesture is reflective of a partnership in which the couple is comprised of two caring companions.

I volunteer to lead a Wii bowling session each week at a local home for seniors. Certainly, there are a number of men and women who are politely genteel in their socialization with one another, but there are several who have gone beyond the winking and smiling stage. I enjoy being with them. They are almost as giddy as junior high school kids at a record hop (if those events still happen any more). Those seniors, many well into their early to mid 90's, have a new reason to rise and shine each morning. They take a serious interest in their exercises and their hygiene. They read and stay current. In other words, they want to stay attractive to that new someone on the second floor. How good is that!

Mutually enjoyable sex is beneficial to achieving quality in life. Sex keeps us active and alive. It is certainly the obvious sign of our health and well-being.

For me, the idea of touching and being touched intimately always puts a smile on my face. It helps me to feel alive, vital and confident. I like being loved and I look forward to my next loving encounter. Do I want to give up my sex life because I have turned 84?

Not "No," but "HELL, NO!"

Elderly Road Trip

....While on a road trip, an elderly couple stopped at a roadside restaurant for lunch. After finishing their meal, they left the restaurant, and resumed their trip.When leaving, the elderly woman unknowingly left her glasses on the table, and she didn't miss them until they had been driving about forty minutes. By then, to add to the aggravation, they had to travel quite a distance before they could find a place to turn around, in order to return to the restaurant to retrieve her glasses. All the way back, the elderly husband became the classic grouchy old man. He fussed and complained, and scolded his wife relentlessly during the entire return drive. The more he chided her, the more agitated he became. He just wouldn't let up one minute. To her relief, they finally arrived at the restaurant. As the woman got out of the car, and hurried inside to retrieve her glasses, the old geezer yelled to her, 'While you're in there, you might as well get my hat and the credit card.'

"Do you remember 20 years ago

A woman awakes during the night to find that her husband-was not in their bed. She puts on her robe and goes downstairs to look for him.She finds him sitting at the kitchen table with a hot cup of coffee in front of him. He appears to be in deep thought, just staring at the wall. She watches as he wiped a tear from his eye and takes a sip of his coffee. "What's the matter, dear?" she whispers as she steps into the room, "Why are you down here at this time of night?" The husband looks up from is coffee, "Do you remember 20 years ago when we were dating, and you were only 16?" he asks solemnly. The wife is touched to tears thinking that her husband is so caring and sensitive. "Yes I do," she replies. The husband paused. The words were not coming easily. "Do you remember when your father caught us in the back seat of my car making love?" "Yes, I remember," said the wife, lowering herself into a chair beside him. The husband continued. "Do you remember when he shoved the shotgun in my face and said, 'Either you marry my daughter, or I will send you to jail for 20 years?' "I remember that too" she replied softly. He wiped another tear from his cheek and said......"I would have gotten out today."

CHAPTER 9

The No Stress Life

If you are feeling stressed over a long period of time, you will definitely be damaging your health

You feel constriction in your chest. Your heart races. You break out in a sweat and may labor to breathe. You feel agitated and may be unable to make simple decisions. If you are being stressed over a long period of time, you will definitely be damaging your health. You can, however, live a longer, happier and healthier life if you remove yourself from the stressful element in your world. That statement is simple enough to comprehend and act upon, unless the stressful element is your spouse or your job. If that is the case, you do have a situation you must deal with.

You may have heard the expression, "If you love your job, you never have to work a day in your life." How true that statement is, and how blessed is the person who said it! Enjoying your associates; earning an adequate income and feeling job satisfaction are work experiences many of us can only dream of. If your work is still on your mind during dinner or when you're watching television; if you toss and turn in bed over the treatment you are receiving from a supervisor or fellow worker; if you find yourself fixated by what tomorrow may bring, you are suffering from anxiety. If that is the case, you just may be entering a minefield of problems which will seriously impact your health.

I've actually heard someone say that they hated their job,

but the only reason they didn't quit was they wanted to see what kind of craziness would occur next. Folks, I'm here to tell you the six o'clock news is filled with craziness, and we have the ability to turn off the set if we choose. We shouldn't have to put ourselves through the hell of being with colleagues who may be seeking power, revenge, or conflict. We shouldn't have to work in a situation of vicious schedules, loud noises and physical endangerment. It may be present a financial hardship, but my advice is to definitely seek to be in a calmer environment. If your spouse is screaming at you, and you are at the point where you no longer can hear his or her voice only a loud obnoxious roar . . . you need to take action NOW!

Many folks want to "fix" their mate. They loved him or her when they first met, even though they were willing to overlook that one little thing that they always found so very irritating. Time passes, and that one little thing becomes a vast warehouse of things that seems to be growing by the day. The main problem that may exist in your marriage might just be that you want to fix the problem while your mate doesn't recognize that a problem even exists. This is when you're going to need to make some very adult decisions.

Counseling could be a first option, but you may need to be prepared for a schism from your mate. Separations are traumatic experiences, but once the dust settles you just might be a happier, healthier you!

Gentle Reader, we were given the gift of life. It is a wonderful gift and we need to cherish it. It is like a wonderful machine that we care for properly. To do so, we need to find that balance in which all facets of it are in tune with one another. If your husband, wife, boss or bowling buddy are simply unbearable to be with any longer, it is not your obligation to fix them. It is your obligation to save yourself.

In order of importance, you're #1. If you take care of that individual, your relationships with your family and peers, friends and neighbors will, or should, become more manageable and beneficial. There are a number of ways you can find this peace you seek. One is simply to become a better listener. One way to achieve this is to occasionally repeat what you believe to be incredulous to the speaker.

"Am I correct here? Are you saying . . ." just be words an individual needs to hear. Sometimes repeating what a person has said acts as a splash of cold water to bring that person back to a harsh reality.

Let me be clear. I am not saying that you as an adult need to divorce yourself from every person or situation you find distasteful. Those negative factors happen in life. I am saying that if you want a long quality lifespan, you need to not be ground down by constant negativity. A person only has so much self-esteem, and others are all too willing to trample it underfoot if they are allowed to do so.

Some good advice might just be to rely heavily on someone you trust greatly . . . a sibling, pastor, long-time best friend. Invite them into your confidence. Lay out what you believe to be your options and seek their counsel. You are not forced to agree with that individual, but you do become aware that someone else has an opinion as to how they might handle your situation. After all, it is your situation.

If there is to be a bottom line for this chapter, it just might be that no one ever really achieves Nirvana in this lifetime. Everyone has their crosses to bear. Everyone has people in their world who cause them consternation. Everyone has people in their workplace who will cause them problems. Your Nirvana comes when you make conscious adult decisions to find and maintain peace of mind.

Be good to yourself. Remember, you are the only you, you have!

GOD'S IMPROVEMENT

A little girl was sitting on her grandfather's lap as he read her a bedtime story. From time to time she would take her eyes off the book and reach up to touch his wrinkled cheek. She was alternately stroking her own cheek, then his again. Finally, she spoke up, "Grandpa, did God make you?" "Yes, sweetheart," he answered, "God made me a long time ago. "Grandpa, did God make me too?" "Yes, indeed, honey," he said, "God made you just a little while ago." Feeling their respective faces again, she observed, "God's getting better at it, isn't he?"

'Sexy Senior Citizen.'

My grandmother has a bumper sticker on her car that says, 'Sexy Senior Citizen.' It's hard to think of my dear old granny in that way. What is she doing? Out entering wet shawl contests? Wheelchair racing? Teeth swapping? Makes me wonder where she got that ten dollar bill she gave me for my birthday. I have become a little older since I saw you last, and a few changes have come into my life since then. Frankly, I have become a frivolous old gal. I am seeing five gentlemen everyday.

As soon as I wake up, Will Power helps me get out of bed. Then I go to see John. Then Charlie Horse comes along, and when he is here he takes a lot of my time and attention. When he leaves, Arthur Ritis shows up and stays the rest of the day. He doesn't like to stay in one place very long, so he takes me from joint to joint. After such a busy day, I'm really tired and glad to go to bed with Ben Gay.

What a life. Oh yes, I'm also flirting with Al Zymer.

Love, Grandma

CHAPTER 10

THE JOY OF VOLUNTEERING

Where else can you have so much fun for so little money!

A great many of my friends volunteer their time and talents, and they do it with loving smiles. They do it all: serve hot meals in soup kitchens, perform clean-up operations, provide rides for the elderly to keep medical appointments and play checkers with a few shut-ins. They actually feel that their hearts by the satisfaction and emotional well-being they derive from their volunteer experiences. You know . . . I'm inclined to believe that they're correct.

Each time I have volunteered, I know how great I felt when after I helped others. The levels of satisfaction and self-esteem I gleaned from those experiences were absolutely second to none.

When I've attempted to explain why I volunteer to some acquaintances, I find them wrinkling their noses and shrugging their shoulders. They respond that they don't understand volunteerism. They just "don't get" volunteers. "Why would I ever want to give my time to do something for nothing," they ask. "My time is my own," they chirp. "I'm retired now. It's time for me to do what I want. Why would I ever think of working with others for absolutely nothing?" Then, they turn and saunter off to go home to DO ABSOLUTELY NOTHING!

Volunteering can, and should, be a healthy part of everyone's life plan. The benefits from volunteering, much like daily physical exercise, is like money in the bank. The purposeful gestures of actions to better the lives of others certainly do impact the provider of the acts possibly as much as the recipients of those same acts. Volunteering   . . . where else can you have so much fun for so little money!

I personally believe that those who volunteer see a marked absence in depression. Moreover, the euphoria felt by volunteers is certainly conducive to overall better health and longevity. Interestingly, vulnerable seniors, i.e. those with chronic health conditions, may benefit the most from volunteering. Those acts of kindness offer volunteers a true feeling of appreciation and vitality. All those acts of kindness can't help but add so much worth to those willing to give of themselves.

Older adults typically volunteer more hours each year than any other age group. These seniors tend to be involved in very purposeful roles within their communities. Younger people may not receive the tremendous health benefits as their senior counterparts. They tend to volunteer out of a sense of obligation or to be involved in the socialization with other young people within the same projects.

Some seniors might balk at volunteering by saying, "I just don't have the time." I contend, "If you want something done . . . ask a busy man to do it." What I mean is people who volunteer tend to find the drive to cram much more living into their days than they ever would have dreamed possible. Further, most everyone can find an excuse not to be involved; the trick is to find a reason to be involved.

Local clubs, churches and organizations generally welcome those who wish to volunteer. Sadly, these same groups are not going to beat the bushes looking for volunteers; they simply don't have the time or resources to do so. Therefore, the responsible adult thing to do is to march into the particular program that may tickle your fancy and state proudly, "I'm here to volunteer. What to you want me to do?"

The volunteer coordinator may not leap out of his chair and over his desk to hug you and thank you for coming through his door that morning, but know in your heart that you are appreciated. Know that the time you take each week to help is necessary. Know that the love you are expressing for your fellow man is warming the hearts of that man and yourself. Also remember, that smile you feel creeping over your lips each time you volunteer is absolutely genuine and never goes out of style.

Here's to all volunteers, those dedicated people who believe in all work and no pay.
  Robert Orben

Volunteers are the only human beings on the face of the earth who reflect this nation's compassion, unselfish caring, patience, and just plain loving one another.
Erma Bombeck

Volunteers are paid in six figures . . . S-M-I-L-E-S.
  Gayla LeMaire

Wherever a man turns he can find someone who needs him.
  Albert Schweitzer

Unselfish and noble actions are the most radiant pages in the biography of souls.
  David Thomas

The breeze, the trees, the honey bees – All volunteers!
  Juliet Carinreap

\

Always remember to forget the troubles that pass your way. But, never forget the blessings that come your way each day.

My Love Dress

"My husband loves me to wear this dress! It makes him happy and it makes me happy. I would appreciate it if you would leave because he will be home from work any minute." The mother-in-law was tired of all this romantic talk and left.

On the way home she thought about the Love Dress. When she got home she got undressed, showered, put on her best perfume and waited by the front door.

Finally her husband got home. He walked in and saw her standing naked by the door.

"What are you doing?" He exclaimed.

"This is My Love Dress." She replied.

"Needs ironing." he said.

"Just doing what you said, Doc:

Morris, an 82 year-old man, went to the doctor to get a physical. A few days later the doctor saw Morris walking down the street with a gorgeous young woman on his arm. A couple of days later the doctor spoke to Morris and said, "You're really doing great, aren't you?" Morris replied, "Just doing what you said, Doc: 'Get a hot mamma and be cheerful.'" The doctor said, "I didn't say that. I said, 'You've got a heart murmur. Be careful.'"

"We had replaced an active, productive lifestyle"

CHAPTER 11

Nothing to do, no place to go

The healthier you are now, the less likely you are to have to deal with costly health problems later

I have known so many seniors who were chained to the same oars as I. We hadn't come to realize that the rut we were in was actually the grave; we merely believed that we temporarily had nothing to do and no places to go. Our health was deteriorating, because we were the cause of our own demise. We spiralled downward blindly. Instead of moving from the work experience that had kept us vital for so many years, we had simply chosen to become isolated. We had replaced an active, productive lifestyle with a passive existence. That existence was an easy trap to fall into. Sadly, we didn't know we were trapped. We didn't feel trapped. And, if we had been told we had become willing victims, we would have denied it.

Some pre-retirees predict that their finances will suffer after retirement, and some retirees say their finances have gotten worse. Only a few pre-retirees think their health will decline in retirement.

Many of us wear rose-colored glasses when we plan for the future, and we need to begin viewing retirement more realistically. When we stop working, our major source of income dries up. And as we get older, it is obvious that our health will deteriorate. So why are so many people underestimating the difficulties of retirement? It is best to plan for these two problems while we are still working and have a good income.

Some two-thirds of Americans do not save enough for retirement. It's time for a reality check. We all need to resolve to save more for retirement and follow through. If you are not saving for retirement right now, it's time to make a plan. It's better to start saving for retirement as early in your career as possible so compound interest will work in your favor. The longer you put off retirement saving, the more difficult it will be to retire comfortably.

Health is a much more difficult issue because there are so many things that we can't control. However, we can focus on the aspects of our health we can do something about. Many American adults are overweight or obese, which is a long-term health risk. Heart disease, strokes, high blood pressure, diabetes, cancer, gout, and many other medical conditions are associated with obesity.

There are also many other lifestyle choices that we can make to maintain good health. Smoking and excessive drinking cause many future health problems such as cancer, liver disease, and diabetes. It's best to moderate our enjoyment of these pleasurable vices to give our future self a better chance at staying healthy. It is important to minimize these health risks as much as we can. This may not be easy, but the healthier you are now, the less likely you are to have to deal with costly health problems later.

A recently published article in Work, Aging and Retirement examined 1,200 service, construction and manufacturing workers. They ranged in age from 52-75. The findings indicated that those without loved ones nearby, as well as those whose health had begun to deteriorate, were at a far greater risk for drug and alcohol abuse than those who stayed active.

Those findings simply document what many of us already have heard over and over again since childhood, "Idle hands are the Devil's workshop." Our parents would toss us out the door early in the morning to work or play, and then gather us up again when the sun was setting. We would be exhausted, but it was a healthy kind of exhaustion. We would clean up, eat, collapse and do it all over again the next day.

I recall the euphoria I felt when I first sold my business. I felt free. I could go anywhere and do anything. I had no responsibilities. Ah, it felt great to be retired. It didn't take long, however, to feel as though I had received an unpardonable lifetime prison sentence. I was trapped in nothingness, and I was drowning. To the casual observer, I appeared to be living the good life, but it was a lie and I knew it. That little voice that all of us know so well was whispering in my ear, and I tried like hell to ignore it.

It's a strange thing about that little voice; it never, ever gives bad advice. Mine was telling me that I was swimming into very deep and very troubled unhealthy waters. It didn't stop there. It tugged mightily on my earlobe saying that I needed to get involved . . . I needed to work out . . . I needed a healthy diet . . . I needed to swim back to the land of the living. So, I did.

Quotes from this chapter

"The findings indicated that those without loved ones nearby, as well as those whose health had begun to deteriorate, were at a far greater risk for drug and alcohol abuse than those who stayed active"

"We hadn't come to realize that the rut we were in was actually the grave; we merely believed that we temporarily had nothing to do and no places to go.

RETIREMENT, A WIFE'S VIEW

A frustrated wife told me the other day her definition of retirement: "Twice as much husband on half as much pay."

And that's how the fight started

One year, a husband decided to buy his mother-in-law a cemetery plot as a Christmas gift...The next year, he didn't buy her a gift. When she asked him why, he replied, "Well, you still haven't used the gift I bought you last year!" And that's how the fight started.

.

"Will you watch us have sexual intercourse?"

A couple, both age 76, went to a sex therapist's office. The doctor asked, "What can I do for you?" The man said, "Will you watch us have sexual intercourse?" The doctor looked puzzled, but agreed. When the couple finished, the doctor said, "There's nothing wrong with the way you have intercourse," and charged them $50. This happened several weeks in a row. The couple would make an appointment, have intercourse with no problems, pay the doctor, then leave. Finally, the doctor asked, "Just exactly what are you trying to find out?" The old man said, "We're not trying to find out anything. She's married and we can't go to her house, I'm married and we can't go to my house. The Holiday Inn charges $90; the Hilton charges $108. We do it here for $50 and I get $43 back from Medicare."

We are now uncertain which one is your husband's.

Mrs. Ward goes to the doctor's office to collect her husband's test results. The lab tech says to her, "I'm sorry, ma'am, but there has been a bit of a mix-up and we have a problem. When we sent the samples from your husband to the lab, the samples from another Mr. Ward were sent as well and we are now uncertain which one is your husband's. Frankly, it is either bad or terrible." "What do you mean?" Mrs. Ward asked. "Well, one has tested positive for Alzheimer's and the other for AIDS. We can't tell which is your husband." "That's terrible! Can we do the test over?" Questioned Mrs. Ward. "Normally, yes. But Medicare won't pay for these expensive tests more than once." "Well, what am I supposed to do now?" "The people at Medicare recommend that you drop your husband off in the middle of town. If he finds his way home, don't sleep with him.

"

Your wife's favorite flower?

While attending a Marriage Weekend, Walter and his wife Ann, listened to the instructor declare, 'It is essential that husbands and wives know the things that are important to each other. 'He addressed the men, 'Can you name and describe your wife's favorite flower? 'Walter leaned over, touched Ann's arm gently and whispered, 'Pillsbury -All-purpose, isn't it?' And thus began Walter's life of celibacy.

When did you graduate?

You've been guilty of looking at others your own age and thinking ...surely I cannot look that old? You may enjoy this short story. While waiting for my first appointment in the reception room of a new dentist, I noticed his certificate, which bore his full name. Suddenly, I remembered that a tall, handsome boy with the same name had been in my high school class some 30 years ago. Upon seeing him, however, I quickly discarded any such thought. This balding, gray-haired man with the deeply lined face was way too old to have been my classmate. After he had examined my teeth, I asked him if he had attended the local high school. "Yes," he replied. "When did you graduate?" I asked. He answered, "In 1971. Why?" "You were in my class!" I exclaimed. He looked at me closely and then asked, "What did you teach?

Romance?

Karl and Milly were lying in bed one night. Carl was falling asleep but Milly was in a romantic mood and wanted to talk. She said, "You used to hold my hand when we were courting."

Wearily Karl reached across, held her hand for a second, and rolled over to try to fall asleep.

A few moments later she said, "Then you used to kiss me."

Mildly irritated, he leaned across, gave her a peck on the cheek and settled back down to sleep.

Thirty seconds later she said, "Then you used to bite my neck."

Angrily, he threw back the bed clothes and got out of bed.

"Where are you going?" she asked.

"To the bathroom to get my teeth," he replied.

I very quietly confided to my best friend that I was having an affair. She turned to me and asked, 'Are you having it catered'? And that, my friend, Is the definition of 'OLD'

CHAPTER 12

PERCEIVED AGE

Age-liars and birthday-deniers

Some of us...are old before our time

Age-liars and birthday-deniers had best learn a thing or two from me, a guy who is young at heart. Blessedly, I feel so much younger than my actual chronological age; I actually smile a great deal, for no apparent reason, at how great I feel.

The Journal of the American Medical Association (JAMA) recently discussed the term perceived age. More accurately stated, the term should be stated as self-perceived age and perceived age. Obviously, the former identifies how we see ourselves. Simply, if we see ourselves as old . . . well, guess what? On the other hand, if we don't consider age as a limiting factor in our lives we would joyously living our lives without laboring under the stigma of getting old.

In her radio ads, Newburyport Attorney Margot Birke asks the question, "How old would you be if you didn't know how old you were?" It is an amazingly simple yet poignant question. Most of us who are adults certainly feel like adults. We do adult things; we drink adult beverages; we watch adult movies; we tell adult jokes, and we understand most of what is happening in life.

Some of us, however, are old before our time. We are way too "early-to-bedders;" we don't stay current with what is happening in the world; we become very set in our ways, unwilling to see the other side in a discussion, and, (this is of utmost importance), we allow ourselves to go downhill because it takes too much work to stay on top of the hill! Those of us who fall into this category have chosen, wittingly or unwittingly, to live as stereo typic "old farts." Our heyday was probably in high school. By 20, we're talking about hobbies, grandchildren and retirement. By 40, we're not just talking the talk, we're walking the walk . . . and now, we're eyeing prime cemetery plots. You can't imagine the hours of fun you would have hanging out with these folks!

Dylan Thomas might have been my kind of guy. He had that certain feistiness needed to keep body and soul together. I love his poem, Do Not Go Gentle into that Good Night. Ponder the first stanza:

> Do not go gentle into that good night,
> Old age should burn and rave at close of day;
> Rage, rage against the dying of the light.

Rage against the dying of the light! Thomas is telling us to live . . . really live, don't just phone it in. While your heart beats, dance . . . sing . . . for God's sake, move!

Okay, okay, let me back up a half step here. Under no circumstances am I advocating that 70-year olds should be looking toward a position as a defensive lineman in the NFL. Don't deny the fact that you have common sense. I am saying that if you are a senior and allow yourself to perceive your own age to be a meaningless factor in how you live, you should perennially be "young at heart." Moreover, if you develop healthier behaviours, your resilience factors will grow stronger . . . you will want to go and do.

Have you ever noticed an old timer who owns a great old car. It could be a MG roadster or a vintage BMW Z3. He takes great care of that vehicle. He oils it, polishes it, cleans the spark plugs, and may even take it out for a drive once a year. All too quickly, the fellow dies and the car is sold to pay for his funeral. What a shame. I'm not talking about the guy, I'm talking about the car! Those babies were meant to zip, and that codger treated it like it was a sacred relic from an Egyptian tomb. For so many years, that guy could have been having a ball motoring top-down across America's heartland. He could have been accompanying Mick Jagger belting out 'Satisfaction.' Instead, he might drop into his garage once a month or so; pull the canvas cover back from his great car; sigh; recover his car; close the door to his garage, and walk back into his house once again. Sadly, the old coot really thought he was living. He was just going through the motions.

That's what I'm talking about here . . . the need to really live. As Thomas said, "Rage against the dying of the light." Ladies and gentlemen, life is not a dress rehearsal. You have one shot to get it all in. I can't imagine a worst death scenario than lying on a bed ruing over what I could have accomplished.

For my money, the best television commercial series has been done by Dos Equis. The commercials feature "The most interesting man in the world." This bearded gentleman seems to have been everywhere and done it all with the most astounding people imaginable. I wonder how many of us quietly grin and nod our heads silently wishing that we could do half of the things done by this Madison Avenue creation. We shrug and create excuses . . . "I would, if I had the money" . . . "I'd love to, but I hate to fly" . . . "I don't read enough and I only speak one language," etc. If we are throwing up excuses, we're doing nothing more than digging deeper the rut we are already in. My thought on the matter is that if you find yourself in rut, stop digging!

As I mentioned, my rut was about to be my grave. I was all but buried in it. My advice to you, gentle reader, is ditch the bad habits, not yourself. Get moving. Find every reason to love yourself. Love others for every reason imaginable. Become productive. Rage! Rage! RAGE!!!

The good news is, you can change your perception of how young you are by keeping yourself in good shape.

Good health is a good attitude. Forget all of those decaying thoughts about people and things that don't matter. Negativity only fosters negativity. Go to the gym, take a long walk, smile at everybody, have more sex. Go out and have some fun, and then go home, have more sex and take a nap. I'd be willing to bet that you'll sleep the night away with a smile on your face.

The Feel-Good Endorphins:

One of the most well-documented reactions that take place after working out is the production of endorphins. These non-additive, feel-good molecules are polypeptides. They bind with neurotransmitters in the brain to reduce pain symptoms. The human body produces at least 20 types of endorphins. These benefit the body in a myriad of ways. Besides relieving pain, endorphins help reduce stress, boost immunity, slow the aging process and create a sense of euphoria

The Internet is a wonderful thing. With little or no expertise, a person can find anything and everything there. The world of research has become so easy, that even I can use it. Recently, I discovered that aging is inevitable (who knew?). How a person ages, however, depends on different factors that can either slow down or speed up the aging process. If a person wants to slow down the process and feel younger to boot, here are some thoughts worth considering:

1. Foods can increase inflammation in the body. These foods play a definite role in obesity, heart disease and cancer. Cutting back on known inflammatory foods may help to stave off many negative health issues. For a healthier living, one should avoid or cut back on: fried and processed foods, sugar, refined carbs (such as: sweets, sodas, and processed white flour), alcohol, salt, corn oil and red meat. Take a few moments. Surf the net. You'll be amazed, and pleasantly so, at the wonderful array of foods you can easily make that are not only good, but good for you.

2. Stay hydrated. Every system in your body depends on

water. Most of us don't drink enough of this vital elixir. Men need about 13 cups of fluids each day. Women require about nine cups. Not drinking enough fluids can result in constipation, balance problems, falls, kidney problems, and a whole litany of other maladies no one wants or needs if they want to lead vital, active lives.

3. Laughing at a funny sitcom or movie not only feels good, it also helps your memory and reduces the stress hormone, cortisol. Find reasons to laugh. Surround yourself with funny folk, and divorce yourself from Gloomy Gusses. Who needs them, anyway?

4. Nitric acid is the magic molecule of wellness. You'll want to keep the fountain of nitric acid flowing.

Three ways to open the floodgates are: meditation, exercise and sex.

Meditation, in the form of prayer, yoga or contemplative alone time seems to work from the inside out to offer the individual a general feeling of well being as well as offering a spiritual tune-up.

Exercise is a structured activity that tones the body, relaxes the mind and increases stamina enough to give the Energizer Bunny a good run for his money.

Sensual events, such as sipping a glass of wine or allowing fine chocolate to melt in your mouth offers the feeling of pleasure.

These are other keys to great health. With your doctor's permission, do them in moderation. Sex, well, it's wonderful, but more about that later.

Quotes from this chapter:

"As I mentioned, my rut was about to be my grave. I was all but buried in it. My advice to you, gentle reader, is ditch the bad habits, not yourself. Get moving. Find every reason to love yourself. Love others for every reason imaginable."

New hearing aid

A man was telling his neighbor, "I just bought a new hearing aid. It cost me four thousand dollars, but it's state of the art It's perfect." "Really," answered the neighbor. "What kind is it?" "Twelve thirty."

Social Security application

A retired gentlemen went into the social security office to apply for Social Security. After waiting in line a long time, he got to the counter. The woman behind the counter asked him for his driver's license to verify his age. He looked in his pockets and realized he had left his wallet at home. He told the woman that he was very sorry but he seemed to have left his wallet at home. "Will I have to go home and come back now?" he asks. The woman says, "Unbutton your shirt." So, he opens his shirt revealing lots of curly silver hair. She says, "That silver hair on your chest is proof enough for me," and she processed his Social Security application. When he gets home, the man excitedly tells his wife about his experience at the Social Security office. She said, "You should have dropped your pants, you might have qualified for disability,

Her Husband of 50 years

"Sugar, why don't you sit down by the table and we'll start supper." said Dorothy to her husband of 50 years. "Sure thing," said her husband settling himself down. "Now darling, would you like the soup first or the salad?" questioned Dorothy. "Umm I guess I'll take the soup" he responded. After a whole meal of one endearing term after another, their guest Bob couldn't contain his curiosity any longer. Bob snuck into the kitchen and asked, "Dorothy do you always talk to your husband like that?" "Bob, I'll be honest with you," Dorothy replied. "It's been five years now, I just can't remember his name, and I am just too embarrassed to ask him!"

Old folks and their problems

A senior citizen said to his eighty-year old buddy: "So I hear you're getting Married?" "Yep!" "Do I know her?" "Nope!" "This woman, is she good looking?" "Not really." "Is she a good cook?" "Naw, she can't cook too well." "Does she have lots of money?""Nope! Poor as a church mouse." "Well then, is she good in bed?" "I don't know." "Why in the world do you want to marry her then?" "Because she can still drive!"

"Do you still have intercourse?"

After the eighty-three year old lady finished her annual physical examination, the doctor said, "You are in remarkable shape for your age, Mrs. Green, but tell me, do you still have intercourse?" "Just a minute, I'll have to ask my husband," she said. She then stepped out into the crowded reception room and yelled out loud: "Bob, do we still have intercourse?" There was then such a hush you could hear a pin drop. Bob, totally unfazed, answered impatiently, "If I told you once, Irma, I have told you a hundred times, what we have is Blue Cross."

Pet Parrot

A man buys a pet parrot and brings him home. But the parrot starts insulting him and gets really nasty, so the man picks up the parrot and tosses him into the freezer to teach him a lesson. He hears the bird squawking for a few minutes, but all of a sudden the parrot is quiet. The man opens the freezer door, the parrot walks out, looks up at him and says, "I apologize for offending you, and I humbly ask your forgiveness."

The man says, "Well, thank you. I forgive you."

The parrot then says, "If you don't mind my asking, what did the chicken do?"

He died of what?

One day I had to be the bearer of bad news when I told a wife that her husband had died of a massive myocardial infarct. Not more than five minutes later, I heard her reporting to the rest of the family that he had died of a "massive internal fart."

CHAPTER 13

HEALTHY AGING

Healthy aging is the continuing ability to find meaning and joy in life.

How you will feel as you get older depends on many things. If you take good care of your body and learn positive ways to deal with stress, you can slow down or even prevent problems that often come with getting older.

It's never too early or too late to change bad habits and start good ones. No matter when you start, a healthy lifestyle can make a difference in how you feel and what you can do.

Just before the funeral services, the undertaker came up to the very elderly widow and asked, 'How old was your husband?' '96,' she replied: 'Two years younger than me' 'So you're 98,' the undertaker commented. She responded, 'Not hardly worth going home, is it?
'

Staying Healthy As You Age

Staying healthy and feeling your best is important at any age and that doesn't change just because you are GETTING OLDER. As we grow older, we experience an increasing number of major life changes, retirement, children leaving home, the loss of loved ones, and physical changes. How we handle and grow from these changes is the key to staying healthy.

I've sure gotten old! I've had two bypass surgeries, a hip replacement, New knees, fought prostate cancer and diabetes I'm half blind, can't hear anything quieter than a jet engine, take 40 different medications that make me dizzy, winded, and subject to blackouts. I have bouts with dementia. Have poor circulation; hardly feel my hands and feet anymore. Can't remember if I'm 85 or 92. Have lost all my friends. But, thank God, I still have my Florida driver's license.

No matter how old you are or how unhealthy you've been in the past, caring for your body has enormous benefits that will help you stay active, sharpen your memory, boost your immune system, manage health problems, and increase your energy. In fact, many older adults report feeling better than ever because they are making more of an effort to be healthy than they did when they were younger.

Preventive measures like healthy eating, exercising, and managing stress can help reduce the risk of chronic disease or injuries later in life. Whether you are generally healthy or are coping with an ongoing injury, disability, or health problem, regular exercise will help you stay physically and mentally healthy and improve your confidence and outlook on life.

An elderly woman decided to prepare her will and told her preacher she had two final requests. First, she wanted to be cremated, and second, she wanted her ashes scattered over Wal-Mart. 'Wal-Mart?' the preacher exclaimed. 'Why Wal-Mart?' 'Then I'll be sure my daughters visit me twice a week.'

Everyone has different ways of experiencing meaning and joy and the activities you enjoy may change over time. Focus on the things you're grateful for. The longer you live, the more you lose. But as you lose people and things, life becomes even more precious. When you stop taking things for granted, you appreciate and enjoy what you have even more.

Know how to prevent sagging? Just eat till the wrinkles fill out.

Acknowledge and express your feelings. You may have a hard time showing emotions, perhaps feeling that such a display is inappropriate and weak. But burying your feelings can lead to anger, resentment, and depression. Don't deny what you're going through. Find healthy ways to process your feelings, perhaps by talking with a close friend or writing in a journal.

It's scary when you start making the same noises as your coffee maker.

Accept the things you can't change. Many things in life are beyond our control. Rather than stressing out over them, focus on the things you can control such as the way you choose to react to problems. Face your limitations with dignity and a healthy dose of humor. Look for the silver lining. As the saying goes, "What doesn't kill us makes us stronger."

These days about half the stuff In my shopping cart says, 'For fast relief.'

When facing major challenges, try to look at them as opportunities for personal growth. Healthy aging means continually reinventing yourself as you pass through land-mark ages such as 60, 70, 80 and beyond. It means finding new things you enjoy, learning to adapt to change, staying physically and socially active, and feeling connected to your community. The truth is that you are stronger and more resilient than you may think.

THOUGHT FOR THE DAY: I don't want to brag or make anyone jealous or anything, but I can still fit into the earrings I wore in high school

Later life can be a time of exciting new adventures if you let it. Taking time to nourish your spirit is never wasted. It's important to find ways to reach out and connect to others, regardless of whether or not you live with a spouse or partner. Having an array of people you can turn to for company and support as you age is a buffer against loneliness, depression, disability, hardship, and loss.

Concerns like: **"Will there enough money now that I'm retired?"** and "What will happen if I get a serious illness or become disabled?" are common in older adults. Stress can have an enormous impact on your health and your quality of life at any age—and even more so as you get older.

AS I AGE, I REALIZE THAT:

1. I talk to myself, because sometimes I need expert advice.

2. Sometimes I roll my eyes out loud.

3. I don't need anger management. I need people to stop pissing me off.

4. My people skills are just fine. It's my tolerance of idiots that needs work.

5. The biggest lie I tell myself is "I don't need to write that down, I'll remember it."

6. When I was a child I thought nap time was punishment. Now it's like a mini vacation.

7. The day the world runs out of wine is just too terrible to think about.

8. Even duct tape can't fix stupid, but it can muffle the sound!

9. Wouldn't it be great if we could put ourselves in the dryer for ten minutes; come out wrinkle-free and three sizes smaller.

10. If God wanted me to touch my toes, he would've put them on my knees.

11. When the kids text me "plz" which is shorter than please. I text back "no" which is shorter than "yes".

12. At my age "Getting lucky" means walking into a room and remembering what I came in there for.

5-LB potato sack in each hand

Younger people try it at their own risk. This is working well for me.

For those of us getting along in years, here is a little secret for building your arm and shoulder muscles. You might want to adopt this three days a week.

Begin by standing straight, with a 5-LB potato sack in each hand. Extend your arms straight out from your sides and hold them there as long as you can. Try to reach a full minute. Relax

After a few weeks, move up to 10-LB. potato sacks, and then 50-LB. potato sacks, and eventually try to get to where you can lift a 100-LB. potato sack in each hand and hold your arms straight out for more than a full minute.

After you feel confident at that level, start putting a couple of potatoes in the bags.

ABOUT GROWING OLDER.

First ~ Eventually you will reach a point when you stop lying about your age and start bragging about it.

Second ~ The older we get, fewer things seem worth waiting in line for.

Third ~ Some people try to turn back their odometers Not me; I want people to know 'why' I look this way. I've traveled a long way, and some of the roads weren't paved.

Fourth ~ When you are dissatisfied and would like to go back to youth, think of Algebra.

Fifth ~ You know you are getting old when every thing either dries up or leaks.

Sixth ~ I don't know how I got over the hill without getting to the top.

Seventh ~ One of the many things no one tells you about aging is that it's such a nice change from being young.

Eighth ~ One must wait until evening to see how splendid the day has been.

Ninth ~ Being young is beautiful, but being old is comfortable and relaxed.

Tenth ~ Long ago, when men cursed and beat the ground with sticks, it was called witchcraft.

Conclusion:

Here are a few more tips to get back to good health

Create your good health plan. Once you know you actually do want to invest time, energy and resources into taking back control of your health and getting on the path of good health. Creating your plan requires you to know what you'd like your body and health to look, feel and be like in about 1-5 years time and then breaking down that vision into monthly goals of nutrition, exercise and anything else needed to get you there.

Get rid of your negative influences. Have you ever tried to improve one part of your life but find that no matter how hard you try, it may not seem to work? It's usually because you haven't cleared out the negative energies or things that are conflicting with it.

. Make a list of things that you are tolerating in your life, things you know you shouldn't do or have but are still doing And slowly cut down and get rid of it.

Drink lots of water. During the course of our sleep, we lose a lot of water during our breathing and so its important that when you get up, you have a big glass of water. The vitality our cells gets from water is very important and useful and will keep our body working in correct order. Without water, our cells starts to wilt just like plants without water.

Eat lots of water-rich content. Our body is made up of about 70% of water just like our planet and so naturally we should consume enough water to keep our body hydrated and enough to recycle our body's capacity every so often. Consume lots of water-rich fruits and vegetables every day. Make a fresh juice every morning with a selection of fruits, and I also try to have at least two big bowls of salad a day –

one at lunch, one at dinner. The simple sugars from fruits are important nutrients and vitamins for our body.

Rest well. Without sleep, our body's clock loses its rhythm and starts to dysfunction, causing poor habits. Rest well and consistently each day. Try to keep your timings consistent so your body can set its routine. If you can't sleep early, get some blindfolds, ear plugs, soothing music, or whatever you need.

Exercise at least 30 minutes a day. If you don't exercise, seriously consider the impacts on your body. Exercise gets your body moving, your blood circulating and your energy in motion. If you work at home or in an office, get up every 30 minutes and walk around. If you have a staircase nearby, run up and down it several times a day. If you can get out for a walk, I highly recommend it for at least 10 minutes once in a day. The great thing is that you can break up your 30 minutes exercise a day into 2-3 segments so you can exercise wherever you are.

Eat your food slower. The Slow Food Movement talks about eating your food slower to aid digestion, heighten the cooking and eating experience and really enjoying your food. I'm in favor for this because of what it can do to your body's digestive system. Research shows that eating slower can make you more fuller and thus you eat less.

Don't overeat. Only eat till you are satisfied. Don't overeat or over-full yourself. Eat with content and till your stomach is satisfied. You can always go and eat something healthy later – and that's better than overeating.

NOT AN OPTION
Decide today which foods for you are NOT an option and then make a firm decision that your life will be so much better without them

.

Stress eating should NOT be an option. Don't do it!

Eating "garbage foods" that will ultimately do more harm than good is NOT an option. Again, don't do it!

Late night munching and too much to drink in an evening is NOT an option. Don't do it!

Fast food hamburger and french fries ...NOT an option. Definitely don't do it!

Check into what foods fall into the "not an option category." You will find there are plenty of foods that should never be eaten again, and you would be perfectly fine.

Try to avoid processed foods and drinks.

This is an option
WASH YOUR HANDS

Wash your hands regularly and disinfect surfaces that are touched by more than one person, particularly if someone in the family is sick. These include doorknobs, refrigerator door handles, microwaves, faucets, and toilet flushers. For electronic devices such as phones, remote controls, game controls, and computer keyboards, wipe with sanitizer cloths or use a product designed for electronics. Computer keyboards can also be covered with a plastic or silicone cover to make cleaning and disinfecting easier. This habit will help prevent you from accidently getting sick from a bacterial disease.

TESTIMONIES

I had asked Annette, what do you do to say healthy?

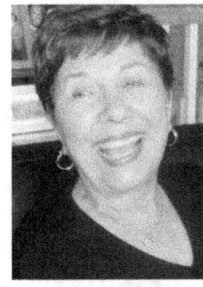

She responded, "I exercise regularly, try to eat a balanced diet, stay active mentally and physically, and laugh a lot.

I asked Jerry, what do you do to stay healthy?

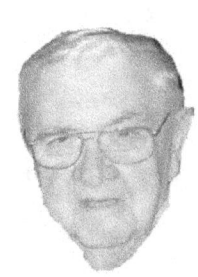

**"Growing old ain't for Sissies.
What don't hoyt it don't woik!**
After retirement in 1995 I knew I had to adopt a healthier life style. I was over weight and had a cadiological problem. I became careful of what I ate, more seafood, greens and etc; less red meats and starches. I started walking along the Seawall. I did approximately ¼ mile and worked it up to 1 mile 3-5 days per week. It took me 3 years, I didn't starve but kept to my general practice and lost 85 pounds and felt a lot better

I keep busy with community activities, work on our house and I always have my great right hand at my side (Marge) with many family activities.

We have been married 61 years, have 5 children, a daughter-in-law, 3 sons-in-law, 8 grandchildren (4-BOYS, 4 GIRLS), 3 Great grandchildren (1 Boy, 2 girls). We have many, many friends all over this beautiful country of ours.

I worked in a profession I loved which took us all over the USA. I am 84 years old and love my wife and family. I can still tell a joke or story and sing a song

What's not to be happy about? The lord God will decide when you have had enough! I have been Blessed!! Jerry D

I asked Debbie, what do you do to stay healthy?

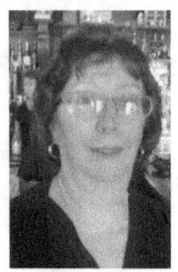

To stay healthy, I have reduced my salt and sugar intake and also try to make sure I don't eat very many processed foods. I also try to walk more. I find it easier to stay on course with making healthier choices by making little changes.

I asked Margaret, what do you do to stay healthy?

Live, love, and laugh a lot, in order to face the challenges of life in a positive way

I asked Richard, what do you do to stay healthy?

Maintain a positive attitude, exercise daily, proper eating, love of family, remember the past and look forward to the future.

I asked Jim, what do you do to stay healthy?

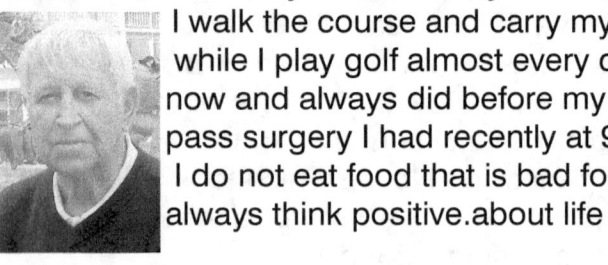

I walk the course and carry my own bag while I play golf almost every day. I do it now and always did before my heart by pass surgery I had recently at 90 years old. I do not eat food that is bad for me and always think positive.about life in general.

"

I asked Tony, what do you do to stay healthy?

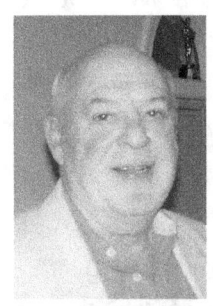 About 20 years ago (1995) my Dr. told me I had diabetes and had to go on a diet. He told me to cut back on things I ate and keep away from sugar.

Over the years after that, even with the pill he gave me I had a hard time keeping my blood sugar levels down. In the morning when I checked my blood level it was around 165 to 185 (should be under100) and my 3 month A one C levels where around 7 to 7.8 and should be under 7. The lower the better.

So over the years I started to change the way (changed food products) I ate. I would try something one day mark down what I was eating and check my blood the next day. If it was high I would eat the same thing but leave out the starch and started to find out that bread potatoes and pasta where the 3 worst things I could eat that would make my blood sugar high.

Even after doing that my blood sugars were still high but lower than before most mornings about 135 to 150 so I started eating my bigger meal in the afternoon still cutting out all bread, potato and pasta. In the evenings I would have only fish or meat with a green vegetable.

This helped even more. .It got my blood sugar levels down under 135 each morning and my 3 month A one C levels around 7 to 7.2.

But a few years ago, I was on the computer and was reading about cinnamon and on the same day about Complete Glucose Support and how it helps people with Diabetes so I got some I take the pills that the Doctor gave me but added the natural pills Glucose and the Cinnamon after each meal. This has helped a lot over the pass 3 or 4 years.

My blood sugar reading in the mornings (as long as I eat no Starch) have been between 80 and 100 and than my 3 months Doctor A one C levels have been between 64 and

70 .

I have also found that if I cheat (like eating a piece of cake at night) and after eating it I walk a mile or so it will not hurt my blood sugar level But that's a SMALL piece of cake and not every night

I asked Jay, what do you do to stay healthy?

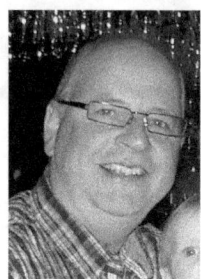

I will be 74 years old when my youngest daughter graduates from high school. That's the best motivation to stay healthy. I'd like to see that graduation day along with a wed ding and meet my future grand children. Right now, I am 58 years old and chasing around a 2 and a 4 years old making sure they are safe and having fun. My wife and I are constantly exhausted but having a fantastic experience each and every day. As older parents, being with our young children keeps us sharp, focused and truly full of joy. Each day is packed with an entire range of emotions due to the many successes and failures; some major, most minor but all entirely significant and passionate.

I asked Bill, what do you do to stay healthy?

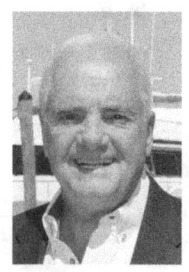

As a former U.S. Marine I was conditioned as a young man to be in shape. I Have maintained a good physical appearance as result of staying in shape. I'm not a gym nut and I never really enjoyed working out, but I manage to do something everyday. Push-ups have always been a staple exercise for Marines and I have continued with push-ups my entire life. At 71 I still do 30 push-ups most days. I keep my stomach in shape with an exercise wheel. It's a tough exercise to work into but once your stomach muscles are conditioned to the exercise wheel it becomes much less difficult and the resulting abs, at any age, make it all worthwhile. For fun and enjoyment I ride a bike along the beach enjoying the sights, getting fresh air, and moving. My three rules for a long healthy life are simple; Eat less; Keep Moving; and Think Happy Thoughts.

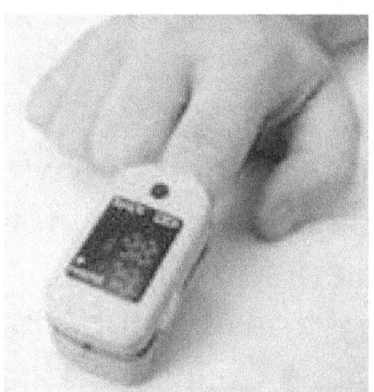

My FRIEND, THE OXIMETER

When I was so very sick, unable to walk and barely able to breathe, I had one constant companion . . . my oximeter. I dare not call it a "friend," because it certainly didn't cheer me much of the time. This little devise has only one function: to measure the amount of oxygen in one's system. Having 95% or better indicates oxygen-rich blood. This is wonderful. My reading was 82%. This B- reading indicated that I had a small amount of oxygen in my lungs. Further, it indicated that I didn't have the energy or vitality to breathe or be active. As I progressed through my daily exercise regimen, my readings rose daily. Exercises and proper nutrition added to my sense of wellbeing. Some months later, I was in fine working order. I said good-bye to my constant companion, and I hope never to see it again!

My hope is that those who have found their way through this book have gained some insight into becoming healthy and maintaining a positive outlook on life. The greatest gift is the gift of life, and the greatest pleasure is the enjoyment of that life for the greatest amount of time. Have fun! Enjoy!
Jack Daly

!

www.ingramcontent.com/pod-product-compliance
Lightning Source LLC
Chambersburg PA
CBHW060424290526
45791CB00002B/862